FAST FACTS

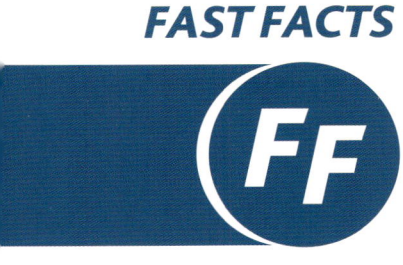

Expert Reviews on Current Research

Psy(
2003–04

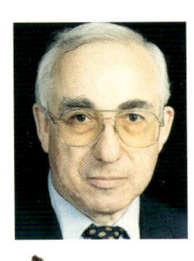

Edited by Malcolm Lader OBE DSc PhD MD
 FRCPsych FMedSci
Emeritus Professor of Clinical Psychopharmacology
Institute of Psychiatry
King's College London
London, UK

This book is as balanced and as up-to-date as we can make it. Ideas for improvements are always welcome: feedback@fastfacts.com

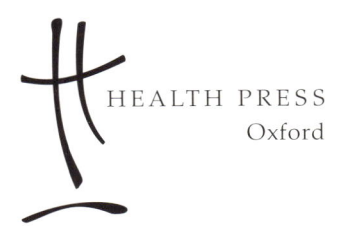

HEALTH PRESS
Oxford

Fast Facts – Psychiatry Highlights 2003–04
First published March 2004

© 2004 Health Press Limited
Health Press Limited, Elizabeth House, Queen Street, Abingdon,
Oxford OX14 3JR, UK
Tel: +44 (0)1235 523233
Fax: +44 (0)1235 523238

Book orders can be placed by telephone or via the website.
For regional distributors or to order via the website, please go to:
www.fastfacts.com
For telephone orders, please call 01752 202301 (UK) or
800 538 1287 (North America, toll free).

Fast Facts is a trademark of Health Press Limited.

All rights reserved. No part of this publication may be reproduced, stored in a retrieval system, or transmitted in any form or by any means, electronic, mechanical, photocopying, recording or otherwise, without the express permission of the publisher.

The publisher and the authors have made every effort to ensure the accuracy of this book, but cannot accept responsibility for any errors or omissions.

Registered names, trademarks, etc. used in this book, even when not marked as such, are not to be considered unprotected by law.

A CIP catalogue record for this title is available from the British Library.

ISBN 1-903734-53-3

Lader, M (Malcolm)
Fast Facts – Psychiatry Highlights 2003–04/
Malcolm Lader

Typesetting and page layout by Zed, Oxford, UK.
Printed by Fine Print (Services) Ltd, Oxford, UK.

Printed with vegetable inks on fully biodegradable and recyclable paper manufactured from sustainable forests.

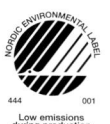

Genetic research in the psychoses
Wolfgang Maier MD — 7

Neurodevelopment and neurodegeneration in schizophrenia
Priya Bajaj MBBS and Tonmoy Sharma MSc MRCPsych — 14

Natural history of bipolar disorder
Alan C Swann MD — 20

Cannabis and psychosis
Zerrin Atakan FRCPsych — 30

Non-pharmacological treatments for anxiety disorders
Jean Cottraux MD PhD — 37

Drug treatment of generalized anxiety disorder
Malcolm Lader OBE DSc PhD MD FRCPsych FMedSci — 43

Recurrent brief depression
David Baldwin FRCPsych — 51

Suicide in custody
Heather Stuart PhD — 56

Post-traumatic stress disorder after earthquakes
Metin Başoğlu MD PhD — 63

Unexplained fatigue symptoms and syndromes
Petros Skapinakis MD MPH PhD and Glyn Lewis FRCPsych PhD — 70

Cancer and mood disorders
Laura K Sherman MD and Michael J Fisch MD MPH — 80

Asperger's syndrome
Jan Blacher PhD and Rachel M Fenning BA — 88

Appendix – Generic and brand names of drugs — 97

Introduction

This is the second *Fast Facts – Psychiatry Highlights*. The first one, published in February 2002, was very well-received, with one reviewer describing it as 'perfect' for those seeking the latest information.[1] It therefore appears to have met the need for busy clinicians to keep abreast of recent developments in the field. This book adopts the same approach as the first, and reviews both academic and more clinical subjects.

The pace of research in psychiatry is undoubtedly accelerating as advances in techniques, such as body imaging, and in theory, such as molecular genetics, are applied to psychiatric problems. These developments have proven to be of immense utility. Furthermore, a more evidence-based approach to therapy has succeeded in winnowing away the chaff, leaving the seed corn for further advances.

Accordingly, *Fast Facts – Psychiatry Highlights 2003–04* has addressed several important topics. A few, such as genetic research in the psychoses, echo the previous book. Others reflect my sense of what is of particular interest to practicing clinicians. Some – such as cannabis and psychosis, suicide in custody, and post-traumatic stress disorder after earthquakes – have proved exceptionally timely, though the topics were chosen before recent widespread media interest.

The contributors were asked to highlight important and changing aspects of their topic, rather than to be comprehensive. All of the experts took time out from their busy professional lives to write these chapters to tight deadlines and I am very grateful to them for their forbearance. I am also grateful to Alison Hillman, Publishing Director of Health Press, for the superbly professional way in which she has accomplished the task of bringing this project to fruition.

Malcolm Lader
Editor

---

[1]'For the reader who is constantly in search of quick facts and the latest information, this book is perfect.' *Doody's Health Sciences Review*, September 2002 (awarded maximum 100 weighted numerical score and 5-star rating).

Genetic research in the psychoses

Wolfgang Maier MD
Department of Psychiatry, University of Bonn, Germany

The genetic basis of psychotic disorders, particularly schizophrenia, was demonstrated nearly a century ago. Since then, twin studies have clearly established that more than 80% of the variance is due to genetic factors, leaving only a marginal role for non-genetic factors.[1] It has been shown that schizophrenia and psychoses belong to the group of genetically complex diseases controlled by multiple disposition genes, rather than by a single causal gene. The search for the genes coding for schizophrenia started two decades ago and, after years of frustration, has recently made major progress.

What has been achieved?

Hypothesis-free approaches to identify disposition genes. In view of our insufficient knowledge of the pathophysiology of the diseases and of appropriate candidate genes, hypothesis-free approaches to finding genes for common diseases have proved useful. Genome-wide linkage analysis in families with multiple affected members has now been established as the first step in identifying candidate regions likely to include disposition genes. In confirmed candidate regions, genetic associations in case-control samples help to localize disposition genes. The power of associations is increased by haplotype analysis.

Linkage analysis to identify candidate regions. Several genome-wide linkage studies in schizophrenia have been performed, but not always with consistent results. Meta-analyses and combined analyses of these genome-wide linkage studies have been instrumental in resolving the inconsistencies. Several candidate regions that had already been proposed from analyses of specific samples have emerged. The candidate regions for psychoses that have been validated are 5q, 3p, 11q, 6p, 1q, 22q, 8p, 20p, 14p, 2p-q and 13q.[2,3]

Detection of first disposition genes. In four candidate regions (6p, 8p, 13q and 22q), positional candidate genes have been successfully explored for associations between DNA sequence variants and schizophrenia. These genes code for dysbindin (6p), neuregulin 1 (NRG-1) (8p), and G72 (13q) which can interact with D-amino acid oxidase (DAAO) and catechol-O-methyltransferase (COMT) (22q).[4] The strength of association observed for single nucleotide polymorphisms (SNPs) was in each case increased by combining SNPs in haplotypes. The risk haplotypes were found to be associated with schizophrenia in several independent replications; non-replications were rare or even revised. The pathogenetic mutation has not yet been identified for any of these genes.

Previously proposed genetic associations discredited. The previously postulated associations between schizophrenia and functional variants of candidate genes coding for 5-hydroxytryptamine$_{2A}$ (5-HT$_{2A}$; serotonin$_{2A}$) and dopamine D$_3$ receptors are now thought to be less strong than initially suspected (odds ratio < 1.2).[5] There is no convincing evidence for dynamic mutations resulting in variation of trinucleotide repeats that were previously proposed to explain anticipation effects (decrease of age at onset from generation to generation).[6]

Establishment of endophenotypes. The phenotype in psychiatric genetic studies is usually defined by diagnosis, which has been refined over recent decades in order to increase reliability and validity, and is now codified as in DSM-IV and ICD-10. It has been argued, however, that genes are not able to read DSM-IV or ICD-10; specific neurobiological vulnerability traits and disease correlates that are more directly related to gene effects have therefore been proposed as alternative phenotypes (endophenotypes).[7] A crucial criterion is the proof of the genetic determination of these traits, and the proof that they share genetic factors with the disorder. It is believed that these traits are influenced by a smaller number of genes, in a simpler manner, than the complex disease.

The most informative type of study for identifying endophenotypes is a discordant twin design study. Such studies have demonstrated that spatial working memory and the volume of prefrontal gray matter meet the endophenotype criteria for schizophrenia.[8,9] Recently, the first endophenotype-based genome scan was published, supporting linkage to region 6p.[10]

What needs to be achieved next?
Functional characterization of identified disposition genes. The first stages of characterizing disposition gene functions have already been accomplished, particularly for NRG-1 which is involved in glial growth and survival. It has also been speculated that glutamatergic transmission defines a common denominator for all identified disposition genes.[11]

Transgenic mouse models are another tool for exploring gene functions. Whereas the NRG-1 gene knock-out mouse reveals some schizophrenia-associated features,[12] a behavioral phenotype of the dysbindin gene knock-out model has so far not been proposed.[13] Knock-out models may not be the most appropriate tool, and modification of gene expression might define more realistic models.

Identification of pathogenetic mutants in known disposition genes. Although disposition genes are proposed, pathogenetic mutants contributing to the manifestation of schizophrenia are completely unknown. Functional characterization of sequence variations are required for this purpose. This might be a difficult task given that each pathogenetic mutant is likely to have only a modest functional effect.

Detection of new disposition genes and their pathogenetic mutants. Genetic investigation of other positional candidates and/or sequencing in order to detect associated DNA sequence variations in the identified candidate regions is in progress in several laboratories.

Highlights in **genetic research in the psychoses** 2003–04

WHAT'S IN?

- Detection of new disposition genes in candidate regions identified by linkage analysis
- Search for pathogenetic mutations and functional characterization of newly detected disposition genes for schizophrenia
- Haplotype instead of single nucleotide polymorphism analysis
- Endophenotype analysis in addition to diagnosis-based linkage analysis
- Genotype–phenotype analysis based on risk haplotypes in identified disposition genes

WHAT'S OUT?

- The hypothesis that linkage analysis does not work for identification of disposition genes in psychoses
- The hypothesis that dynamic mutations/unstable DNA contribute substantially to the causation of schizophrenia
- The idea that there are major genes for schizophrenia
- The proposition that phenotypes defined by diagnosis will prohibit the detection of disposition genes

This search for pathogenetic variants is facilitated by highly informative marker systems, such as SNPs, and haplotype analysis, which is currently developing rapidly. Genome-wide haplotype maps and haplotype tagging maps will provide powerful and cost-efficient strategies for identification of disease genes.[14]

Genome-wide association studies. The hypothesis-free search for predisposing genes for complex disorders has until now been based on linkage studies, but this strategy is limited by the low power for detection of modest-to-small gene effects.[15] Association studies are more powerful in this respect, but genome-wide association studies have not been feasible until recently, because linkage disequilibrium (association) is maintained across only small distances along the genome. Association studies require at least 500 000 equidistant polymorphic markers for a genome-wide coverage, and the SNP marker system, with 2–3 million biallelic polymorphisms, offers this possibility. In addition, the use of genomic controls will help to exclude stratification artifacts.[16] The very large case-control samples necessary for this purpose are currently being recruited in many centers.

Epigenetic studies. All complex, non-mendelian disorders reveal a series of characteristics that suggest epigenetic factors operate in addition to DNA sequence variations. Such epigenetic factors are partly heritable modifications of gene expression (e.g. DNA methylation and stability of the chromatin structure).

Pre- and post-natal stochastic and environmental events may influence the epigenetic profile and accumulate over time, resulting in over- or under-expression of critical disorder-related genes. These mechanisms might explain the incomplete penetrance and dissimilarities of clinical profiles among genetically identical twins and the variation of age at onset of vulnerable subjects later in life. Strong evidence for universal intra- and inter-individual epigenetic variations of relevant genes has recently been described for monozygotic twins with and without schizophrenia.[17] Investigating the epigenetic regulation of genes in parallel with DNA sequence variations may be a fruitful approach in the search for genetic causes of complex disorders.

Pharmacogenetic studies. Differing responses to neuroleptics (both beneficial and adverse) reveal a strong inter-individual variation, which is likely to be driven by the inter-individual variation of DNA sequence. Pharmacogenetic studies try to identify predictive genetic markers in order to optimize the choice of treatment for a specific patient and to establish individualized therapy. Functional candidate gene variants are of particular interest as they may offer insights into mechanisms of action. This line of research is supplemented by neuroimaging studies with appropriately tailored ligands that have differential binding because of genetic variations. So far, only a very few postulated genotype/drug effect associations have been confirmed by replication or meta-analysis (e.g. D_3-receptor gene polymorphism and tardive dyskinesia).[18] Genetic analyses in large cohorts of patients receiving standardized long-term treatment are needed to identify the presumed multiple predictive DNA variants, each of which may have only a small effect.

References

1. McGuffin P, Asherson P, Owen M, Farmer A. The strength of the genetic effect. Is there room for an environmental influence in the aetiology of schizophrenia? *Br J Psychiatry* 1994;164:593–9.

2. Badner JA, Gershon ES. Meta-analysis of whole-genome linkage scans of bipolar disorder and schizophrenia. *Mol Psychiatry* 2002;7:405–11.

3. Lewis MC, Levinson DF, Wise LH et al. Genome scan meta-analysis of schizophrenia and bipolar disorder. Part II: Schizophrenia. *Am J Hum Genet* 2003;73:34–48.

4. O'Donovan MC, Williams NM, Owen MJ. Recent advances in the genetics of schizophrenia. *Hum Mol Genet* 2003;12(suppl 2):R125–33.

5. McGuffin P, Tandon K, Corsico A. Linkage and association studies of schizophrenia. *Curr Psychiatry Rep* 2003;5:121–7.

6. Fortune MT, Kennedy JL, Vincent JB. Anticipation and CAG*CTG repeat expansion in schizophrenia and bipolar affective disorder. *Curr Psychiatry Rep* 2003; 5:145–54.

7. Gottesman II, Gould TD. The endophenotype concept in psychiatry: etymology and strategic intentions. *Am J Psychiatry* 2003;160:636–45.

8. Cannon TD, Huttunen MO, Lonnqvist J et al. The inheritance of neuropsychological dysfunction in twins discordant for schizophrenia. *Am J Hum Genet* 2000;67:369–82.

9. Cannon TD, Thompson PM, van Erp TG et al. Cortex mapping reveals regionally specific patterns of genetic and disease-specific gray-matter deficits in twins discordant for schizophrenia. *Proc Natl Acad Sci USA* 2002;99:3228–33.

10. Hallmayer JF, Jablensky A, Michie P et al. Linkage analysis of candidate regions using a composite neurocognitive phenotype correlated with schizophrenia. *Mol Psychiatry* 2003;8:511–23.

11. Harrison PJ, Owen MJ. Genes for schizophrenia? Recent findings and their pathophysiological implications. *Lancet* 2003;361:417–19.

12. Stefansson H, Sigurdsson E, Steinthorsdottir V et al. Neuregulin 1 and susceptibility to schizophrenia. *Am J Hum Genet* 2002;71:877–92.

13. Li W, Zhang Q, Oiso N et al. Hermansky–Pudlak syndrome type 7 (HPS-7) results from mutant dysbindin, a member of the biogenesis of lysosome-related organelles complex 1 (BLOC-1). *Nat Genet* 2003;35:84–9.

14. Johnson GCL, Esposito L, Barratt BJ et al. Haplotype tagging for the identification of common disease genes. *Nat Genet* 2001;29:233–7.

15. Risch NJ. Searching for genetic determinants in the new millennium. *Nature* 2000;405:847–56.

16. Devlin B, Roeder K. Genomic control for association studies. *Biometrics* 1999;55:997–1004.

17. Petronis A, Gottesman II, Kan P et al. Monozygotic twins exhibit numerous epigenetic differences: clues to twin discordance? *Schizophr Bull* 2003;29:169–78.

18. Basile VS, Masellis M, Potkin SG, Kennedy JL. Pharmacogenomics in schizophrenia: the quest for individualized therapy. *Hum Mol Genet* 2002;11:2517–30.

Neurodevelopment and neurodegeneration in schizophrenia

Priya Bajaj MBBS and **Tonmoy Sharma** MSc MRCPsych

Clinical Neuroscience Research Centre, Dartford, Kent, UK

Schizophrenia, by definition, implies a mental condition characterized by schism, disintegration or dysconnectivity. Almost a century ago, Bleuler expressed it as follows: "the thousands of associations guiding our thought are interrupted by this disease in an irregular way here and there, sometimes more, sometimes less. The thought processes as a result, become strange and illogical, and the associations find new paths".[1]

Neurodevelopmental model

The neurodevelopmental model hyothesizes that schizophrenia is caused by the interaction between genetic and environmental events during critical early periods in neuronal growth which may negatively influence the way the nerve cells are laid down, differentiated and selectively culled by apoptosis.[2]

The neurodevelopmental hypothesis was proposed in the 1980s[3,4] and has been supported by several pieces of evidence, including:[5]
- increased frequency of obstetric complications surrounding the birth of patients with schizophrenia
- the presence of minor physical anomalies
- the presence of neurological, cognitive and behavioral dysfunction long before illness onset
- a course and outcome of the illness that is incompatible in most cases with a degenerative illness
- the stability of brain structural measures over time
- the absence of postmortem evidence of neurodegeneration.

However, the evidence to support the neurodevelopmental hypothesis remains circumstantial, at least in part, because normal human brain development is not amenable to direct investigation.

In fact, during the first half of this century, schizophrenia was described as the 'graveyard of neuropathologists' as a result of the frustrating and inconsistent search for brain abnormalities associated with this illness.

MRI has clearly established that the temporal lobe, the temporal lobe gray matter, and specific mesial and lateral temporal lobe structures are reduced in size by 10–15% in patients with schizophrenia. Subtle volumetric reductions have been demonstrated in widespread cortical areas, including the frontal and parietal secondary association areas.[6] The ventriculomegaly and reduced volumes of the temporal lobe structures were shown not to worsen with time in earlier studies, suggesting that schizophrenia, in contrast to Alzheimer's disease, is not due to a true progressive, degenerative illness. However there is some recent evidence of brain volume changes over time.[5]

The results of postmortem morphometric studies of brains from schizophrenic patients are convincingly consistent with those of in-vivo imaging studies. In addition to the findings outlined above, thinner parahippocampal cortices, reduced hippocampal volumes, smaller thalami[7] and an increased prevalence of cavum septum pellucidum have been reported in schizophrenic brains.[8]

One crucial, relatively consistent observation is the lack of gliosis in schizophrenia. Since proliferation of glial cells is seen in most degenerative brain conditions and encephalopathies that arise after birth, this negative result is more consistent with events that predate the responsivity of glial cells to injury, which is before the third trimester of gestation. Also, abnormalities in the cellular architecture have been found in the hippocampus and the prefrontal cortex. A reduced volume of neuronal projections and number of dendritic spines has been reported, which may contribute significantly to abnormalities in cortical activation and cognitive deficits.[9]

Functional neuroimaging

Various imaging techniques such as positron emission tomography (PET), single photon emission computed tomography (SPECT) and, more recently, functional MRI have been used to look at changes in

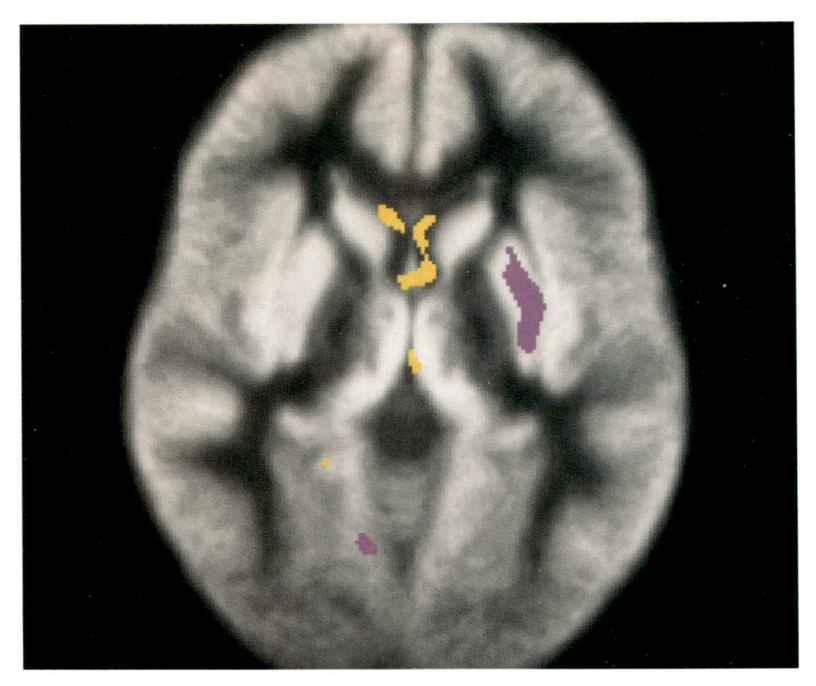

Figure 1 Structural imaging scan of a patient with schizophrenia, showing areas of tissue loss.

regional neural activity and explore brain regions that may be dysfunctional in schizophrenia (Figure 1). However, the most consistent finding to date is reduced activation of the prefrontal cortex (hypofrontality,[10] left prefrontal cortex[11]), although other regions such as the temporal lobes have also been implicated. It is increasingly being recognized that schizophrenia is an illness of disturbed cortical networks.[12]

Neurodegenerative model

The existence of neurodegeneration is the subject of debate in schizophrenia research. The neurodegenerative school points to the typical behavioral and cognitive downhill course of schizophrenic disorders, and cautions that our technical inability to image progressive cell death does not mean that disruptive brain processes do not occur.

> **Highlights in neurodevelopment and neurodegeneration in schizophrenia 2003–04**
>
> **WHAT'S IN?**
> - Neurodegenerative hypothesis
> - Progressive changes in volume measurements in structural MRI
> - Progressive sulcal CSF volume enlargement
> - Dynamic pathophysiological model
> - Cortical network dysfunction
>
> **WHAT'S OUT?**
> - Non-progressive neuropathological changes

Furthermore, neuronal cell bodies may not die. It has been postulated that there may be structural changes in dendrites and axons, impairment in protein metabolism, decrease in the size of neurons and disruptions of synaptic architecture, including maldistributed receptors with consequently disturbed function.[13] It is suggested that these various changes may occur as a result of:[14]

- alterations in membrane phospholipids that lead to cell damage over time
- free radicals acting as toxins in those brains that have poor antioxidant defense.

Perhaps the most robust method to ascertain whether there are progressive neural changes in schizophrenia is by within-subject longitudinal neuroimaging studies. Recent studies of first-episode patients, those with chronic disease and patients with childhood-onset schizophrenia seem to provide increasingly convergent evidence that structural brain deficits in schizophrenia are progressive.[13] In a recent large study of 73 subjects using serial high-resolution MRI, accelerated enlargements in cortical sulcal CSF spaces were found early in the course of schizophrenia. The patients showed a progressive reduction in frontal lobe volume over time and a reciprocal increase in frontal lobe CSF volume, which occurred at a more rapid rate than in controls.[6]

Limitations of current research methods

Although various structural brain abnormalities have been demonstrated in schizophrenia, it is difficult to ascertain their onset. Currently, there are no efficient methods to identify and study individuals before overt onset of the disease. Healthy relatives of schizophrenic patients have brain volumes that are intermediate between patients and controls, suggesting that structural brain abnormalities may be a vulnerability marker.[15,16]

Longitudinal neuroimaging studies are particularly challenging to perform, given the difficulties in getting patients and control subjects to return for additional MRI scans. Furthermore, the rapid advances in neuroimaging technology complicate comparisons of the scans obtained. In addition, most studies have relatively small sample sizes and often use images of non-contiguous slices that provide poor anatomic resolution.[9] Some studies have shown the effects of cortical network dysfunction to be reversed by atypical antipsychotics.[10]

Finally, the pathogenic changes and mechanisms underlying the progressive reduction in frontal lobe volume in schizophrenia still remain unexplained, challenging neurobiologists and inviting new pathophysiological models.[14]

References

1. Kotrla KJ, Sater AK, Weinberger DR. Neuropathology, neurodevelopment, and schizophrenia. In: Keshavan MS, Murray RM, eds. *Neurodevelopment and Adult Psychopathology.* Cambridge: Cambridge University Press, 1997:187–98.

2. Nadri C, Kozlovsky N, Agam G. Schizophrenia, neurodevelopment and glycogen synthase kinase-3. *Psychiatry Res* 2003;122:89–97.

3. Marenco S, Weinberger DR. The neurodevelopmental hypothesis of schizophrenia: following a trail of evidence from cradle to grave. *Dev Psychopathol* 2000;12:501–27.

4. Weinberger DR. Implications of normal brain development for the pathogenesis of schizophrenia. *Arch Gen Psychiatry* 1987;44:660–9.

5. Ho B, Andreasen N, Nopoulos P et al. Progressive structural brain abnormalities and their relationship to clinical outcome. *Arch Gen Psychiatry* 2003;60:585–94.

6. Fannon D, Chitnis X, Doku V et al. Features of structural brain abnormality detected in early first episode psychosis. *Am J Psychiatry* 2000;157:1829–34.

7. Ettinger U, Chitnis XA, Kumari V et al. Magnetic resonance imaging of the thalamus in first-episode psychosis. *Am J Psychiatry* 2001;158:116–18.

8. Wright IC, Ellison ZR, Sharma T et al. Mapping of grey matter changes in schizophrenia. *Schizophr Res* 1999;35:1–14.

9. McCarley RW, Wible CG, Frumin M et al. MRI anatomy of schizophrenia. *Biol Psychiatry* 1999;45:1099–1119.

10. Honey GD, Bullmore ET, Soni W et al. Differences in frontal cortical activation by a working memory task following substitution of risperidone for typical antipsychotic drugs in patients with schizophrenia. *Proc Natl Acad Sci* 1999;96:13432–7.

11. Russell TA, Rubia K, Bullmore ET et al. Exploring the social brain in schizophrenia: left prefrontal underactivation during mental state attribution. *Am J Psychiatry* 2000;157:2040–2.

12. Sharma T. Insights and treatment options for psychiatric disorders guided by functional MRI. *J Clin Invest* 2003;112:10–18.

13. Lieberman JA. Is schizophrenia a neurodegenerative disorder? A clinical and neurological perspective. *Biol Psychiatry* 1999;46:729–39.

14. Weinberger DR, McClure RK. Neurotoxicity, neuroplasticity and magnetic resonance imaging morphometry. What is happening in the schizophrenic brain? *Arch Gen Psychiatry* 2002;59:553–8.

15. Sharma T, Lancaster E, Lee D et al. Brain changes in schizophrenia. A volumetric MRI study of families affected with schizophrenia – The Maudsley Family Study 5. *Br J Psychiatry* 1998;173:132–8.

16. Schulze K, McDonald C, Frangou S et al. Hippocampal volume in familial and nonfamilial schizophrenic probands and their unaffected relatives. *Biol Psychiatry* 2003;53:562–70.

Natural history of bipolar disorder

Alan C Swann MD
Department of Psychiatry, University of Texas Medical School at Houston, USA

Bipolar disorder is usually a lifelong, chronic or recurrent illness. When subsyndromal forms of mania are included, it affects about 6.5% of the population.[1] Bipolar disorder is a highly familial illness which usually begins in adolescence or early adulthood. It is associated with increased susceptibility to other serious medical and psychiatric disorders, and with substantial mortality from suicide (Table 1). This chapter reviews recent information concerning the natural history of bipolar disorder, and the discussion will, of necessity, include patients receiving a variety of treatments. However, in an attempt to focus on the natural history of the illness, controlled treatment studies or studies in which pharmacological response was a primary outcome are not discussed.

Onset of illness

First episode. The onset of bipolar disorder typically occurs between 15 and 25 years.[2] Onset may be earlier and prepubertal onset is more common in patients born since 1940.[3] Age of onset is similar in affected siblings[2] and is earlier in patients with a family history of bipolar disorder.[3]

The first episode of bipolar disorder is usually depression.[4,5] However, because identification of mania or hypomania is necessary for diagnosis, patients with initial depressive episodes may go undiagnosed for years and may be treated inappropriately. Data on the consequences of this diagnostic delay are mixed; one study found no associated differential morbidity,[6] while another found an association with poor social function, more frequent hospitalizations and greater likelihood of suicidal behavior.[7]

At the time of first mania, other symptomatic psychiatric

TABLE 1

Central features of bipolar disorder

Onset
- Usually adolescent or early adulthood; prepubertal onset possible
- Prodromes may precede onset of specific episodes
- Early onset may be associated with a higher risk of bipolar disorder in family members and a greater severity of illness

Recurrence
- Susceptible to depressive, manic or mixed episodes
- Frequency and/or severity of episodes may accelerate

Complications
- Susceptibility to substance abuse
- Susceptibility to anxiety disorders
- Susceptibility to psychosis

Functional impairments
- Impaired occupational and social function

Mortality
- Suicide rate increased at least 20-fold
- Increased all-cause mortality

disorders are generally already present; for example, there may be depression or schizophrenia[8] and, in adolescents, a history of attention deficit disorder.[9]

Prepubertal bipolar disorder. Diagnostic standards for bipolar disorder were developed for adults rather than children and, as a result, the extent and definition of prepubertal illness has been controversial. Careful study of the phenomenology of early-onset bipolar disorder, taking developmental considerations into account, has demonstrated that prepubertal bipolar disorder appears to be a valid clinical entity with specific differentiating features, familial

traits, treatment response and a characteristic course, as follows.[10]
- There is a prominent family history of early onset and there appears to be a greater risk of bipolar disorder in relatives.[11,12]
- Rather than classically organized episodes, the clinical picture is one of prominent mixed states together with chronicity, psychosis and rapid or continuous cycling, resembling severe bipolar disorder in adults.[13]
- Within these disorganized episodes are the classic core symptoms of depression (anhedonia, hopelessness, suicidal thoughts) and/or mania (elation, grandiosity, flight of ideas/racing thoughts, decreased need for sleep, hypersexuality), which are distinct from the less goal-directed hyperactivity, non-specific irritability, accelerated speech and distractibility that are present in attention deficit disorders.[13-15]
- Coexistent or pre-existent conduct disorder[16] or attention deficit disorders are usually present,[17] and the symptoms of bipolar disorder and the disruptive behavior disorder are essentially additive.
- Outcome at 2 years is poor: 65% of patients recover after an average of 36 weeks of treatment, and 55% relapse at an average of 28.6 weeks after recovery.[14]

Offspring of parents with bipolar disorder appear to be at high risk of developing bipolar or other psychiatric disorders.[18]

Prodromes of first episodes. There may be early warnings of the onset of bipolar disorder. A retrospective study of children showed that the principal components of early behavior were irritability/dyscontrol (impulsivity, aggression, decreased attention span, tantrums, hyperactivity), which appeared at 1–6 years of age in subjects who ultimately developed bipolar disorder, while depression, mania and psychosis tended not to appear until the age of 6–12 years.[19]

Course of illness
Relationship between onset and subsequent course. The course of the illness was worse in those patients whose first episode was

depressive, with more severe mood instability and suicidal tendencies. However, delay in initiating appropriate treatment, or early treatment with antidepressants but not with mood-stabilizing agents, may account for this difference.[5] 'Atypical' unipolar patients have been shown to differ from 'non-atypical' unipolar patients, but not from patients with bipolar II disorder in terms of age of onset, incidence of mixed depression (three or more manic symptoms during a depressive episode) and family history.[20] Atypical features were related to early onset (during or before adolescence), which itself appears to be associated with a severe course of illness, including rapid-cycling or severe mood lability, and concomitant axis I disorders including substance use disorders.[21]

Recurrence is the hallmark of bipolar disorder. However, life charting can enhance the effectiveness of treatment and quality of life through improved communication with the patient, understanding of the course of illness, and anticipation of episodes and their prodromes.[22] Life charting of 258 patients over 1 year revealed that they spent 30% of their time depressed and about 10% of the time manic; almost two-thirds of patients had more than three episodes over the year.[23]

In the German centers of the Stanley Foundation Bipolar Network, recurrence was associated with additional axis I diagnoses, more treatment with mood-stabilizing and/or antipsychotic agents, and an increased rate of suicide attempts.[24] Prospective weekly life charting (for an average of 13.4 years) of 86 patients with bipolar II disorder revealed that they were symptomatic on 53.9% of occasions, and that symptoms were depressive for about 90% of the time. A long index episode, a positive family history of bipolar disorder and poor previous social function were all associated with chronicity of illness.[25]

The course of bipolar disorder also appears to be influenced by reproductive events. A small study found that disease onset occurred within 1 year of menarche in 25 of 50 women with bipolar disorder.[26] Of the 30 women who had children, 20 had

> ### *Highlights in* **natural history of bipolar disorder** *2003*
>
> **WHAT'S EMERGING?**
>
> - Vulnerability to affective and behavioral instability and to recurrence, rather than affective episodes themselves, as the true hallmark of the illness
> - Presence of prepubertal illness with strong familial traits, and a severe presentation and course
> - Prodromal symptoms and psychiatric problems before the first episode of depression or mania
> - Depression as the first affective episode and the dominant source of impairment for most patients
> - Comorbidities, especially anxiety and substance use disorders, as expressions of severe underlying pathophysiology
> - Suicidal behavior as an expression of illness severity, also associated with severe affective instability and comorbid disorders
> - Extreme variability in the course of illness, with little relationship between the severity of a specific episode and the severity of the overall course of illness

postpartum episodes, which were predicted by depressive symptoms during pregnancy and by depressive episodes after earlier pregnancies.

Rapid-cycling is formally defined as at least four episodes over 12 months, but the term can describe a wide variety of cycle lengths ranging from months to days. The long-term course of rapid-cycling is still a matter of debate and is likely to remain so as long as the definition remains so vague. Follow-up of 109 patients with rapid-cycling over 2–26 years (mean 11 years) revealed a mixed outcome: 33% achieved complete remission, 40% continued rapid-cycling (6 of these 44 patients committed suicide), 14% experienced reduced severity and 13% reverted to 'long-cycling'.[27] The onset of

> **WHAT'S NEEDED?**
> - Better understanding of prepubertal depression and mania, and their relationship to bipolar disorder in adults
> - Tools for early prediction of the course of illness, treatment response and the likelihood of complicating disorders
> - Tools for predicting the likelihood of relapse in any patient throughout the life cycle

> **WHAT'S NEEDED MOST?**
> - Understanding of the pathophysiology of the lifelong risk for recurrence of affective episodes and related problems
> - A means for diagnosing bipolar disorder reliably without having to wait for episodes of mania or hypomania

rapid-cycling appeared to be associated with antidepressant or other treatments in 88%; in the other 12% it was spontaneous.

Late-onset bipolar disorder. It remains controversial whether late-onset bipolar disorder differs from early-onset bipolar disorder with respect to the role of genetic compared with other medical causes. Among 6182 patients in Western Australia with primary or secondary diagnoses of bipolar disorder, 8% experienced onset after 65 years of age. Only a small fraction (2.8%) had organic disorders, and there were no large clinical differences between the conventional and late-onset groups.[28]

Screening instruments may be valuable for detecting patients who merit more careful evaluation for bipolar disorder. The Mood

Disorders Questionnaire, which was developed for this purpose, can identify those who will experience more work problems, more social and leisure problems, and more family problems.[29]

Comorbidities. Bipolar disorder confers increased risk of other psychiatric illness, especially substance use and anxiety disorders, as well as non-psychiatric conditions such as migraine and atherosclerotic heart disease. A review of family studies of bipolar disorder suggests that these comorbidities generally result from multiple expressions of the underlying pathophysiology, reflecting greater severity of the underlying illness.[30] Accordingly, patients with coexisting panic disorder had more depressions, more suicidal behavior and a longer time before remission than those without panic disorder.[31]

Mortality

Untreated bipolar disorder is associated with increased mortality, regardless of gender or age. Comorbidities increase the likelihood of suicide attempts. Substance abuse doubled the risk of suicide attempts in 336 subjects.[32]

Among 406 patients followed prospectively for up to 22 years, most excess mortality was due to suicide and circulatory disorders. Treatment, with combinations of lithium, other mood stabilizers, antidepressants and antipsychotic agents, reduced the likelihood of suicide even though treated patients were more severely ill.[33]

References

1. Judd LL, Akiskal HS. The prevalence and disability of bipolar spectrum disorders in the US population: re-analysis of the ECA database taking into account subthreshold cases. *J Affect Disord* 2003;73:123–31.

2. Bellivier F, Golmard JL, Rietschel M et al. Age at onset in bipolar I affective disorder: further evidence for three subgroups. *Am J Psychiatry* 2003;160:999–1001.

3. Chengappa KN, Kupfer DJ, Frank E et al. Relationship of birth cohort and early age at onset of illness in a bipolar disorder case registry. *Am J Psychiatry* 2003; 160:1636–42.

4. Hirschfeld RM, Lewis L, Vornik LA. Perceptions and impact of bipolar disorder: how far have we really come? Results of the national depressive and manic-depressive association 2000 survey of individuals with bipolar disorder. *J Clin Psychiatry* 2003;64:161–74.

5. Perugi G, Micheli C, Akiskal HS et al. Polarity of the first episode, clinical characteristics, and course of manic depressive illness: a systematic retrospective investigation of 320 bipolar I patients. *Compr Psychiatry* 2000;41:13–18.

6. Baldessarini RJ, Tondo L, Hennen J. Treatment-latency and previous episodes: relationships to pretreatment morbidity and response to maintenance treatment in bipolar I and II disorders. *Bipolar Disord* 2003;5:169–79.

7. Goldberg JF, Ernst CL. Features associated with the delayed initiation of mood stabilizers at illness onset in bipolar disorder. *J Clin Psychiatry* 2002;63:985–91.

8. Daniels BA, Kirkby KC, Mitchell P et al. Heterogeneity of admission history among patients with bipolar disorder. *J Affect Disord* 2003; 75:163–70.

9. Soutullo CA, DelBello MP, Ochsner JE et al. Severity of bipolarity in hospitalized manic adolescents with history of stimulant or antidepressant treatment. *J Affect Disord* 2002;70:323–7.

10. Biederman J, Mick E, Faraone SV et al. Current concepts in the validity, diagnosis and treatment of paediatric bipolar disorder. *Int J Neuropsychopharmacol* 2003;6: 293–300.

11. Faraone SV, Glatt SJ, Tsuang MT. The genetics of pediatric-onset bipolar disorder. *Biol Psychiatry* 2003;53:970–7.

12. Somanath CP, Jain S, Reddy YC. A family study of early-onset bipolar I disorder. *J Affect Disord* 2002;70: 91–4.

13. Craney JL, Geller B. A prepubertal and early adolescent bipolar disorder-I phenotype: review of phenomenology and longitudinal course. *Bipolar Disord* 2003;5: 243–56.

14. Geller B, Craney JL, Bolhofner K et al. Two-year prospective follow-up of children with a prepubertal and early adolescent bipolar disorder phenotype. *Am J Psychiatry* 2002; 159:927–33.

15. Geller B, Zimerman B, Williams M et al. DSM-IV mania symptoms in a prepubertal and early adolescent bipolar disorder phenotype compared to attention-deficit hyperactive and normal controls. *J Child Adolesc Psychopharmacol* 2002;12:11–25.

16. Wozniak J, Monuteaux M, Richards J et al. Convergence between structured diagnostic interviews and clinical assessment on the diagnosis of pediatric-onset mania. *Biol Psychiatry* 2003;53: 938–44.

17. Galanter CA, Carlson GA, Jensen PS et al. Response to methylphenidate in children with attention deficit hyperactivity disorder and manic symptoms in the multimodal treatment study of children with attention deficit hyperactivity disorder titration trial. *J Child Adolesc Psychopharmacol* 2003;13:123–36.

18. Chang K, Steiner H, Dienes K et al. Bipolar offspring: a window into bipolar disorder evolution. *Biol Psychiatry* 2003;53:945–51.

19. Fergus EL, Miller RB, Luckenbaugh DA et al. Is there progression from irritability/dyscontrol to major depressive and manic symptoms? A retrospective community survey of parents of bipolar children. *J Affect Disord* 2003;77:71–8.

20. Benazzi F. Is there a link between atypical and early-onset 'unipolar' depression and bipolar II disorder? *Compr Psychiatry* 2003;44:102–9.

21. Carter TD, Mundo E, Parikh SV, Kennedy JL. Early age at onset as a risk factor for poor outcome of bipolar disorder. *J Psychiatr Res* 2003;37:297–303.

22. Wittchen HU, Mühlig S, Pezawas L. Natural course and burden of bipolar disorders. *Int J Neuropsychopharmacol* 2003;6:145–54.

23. Post RM, Denicoff KD, Leverich GS et al. Morbidity in 258 bipolar outpatients followed for 1 year with daily prospective ratings on the NIMH life chart method. *J Clin Psychiatry* 2003;64:680–90.

24. Dittmann S, Biedermann NC, Grunze H et al. The Stanley Foundation Bipolar Network: results of the naturalistic follow-up study after 2.5 years of follow-up in the German centres. *Neuropsychobiology* 2002;46(suppl 1):2–9.

25. Judd LL, Akiskal HS, Schettler PJ et al. A prospective investigation of the natural history of the long-term weekly symptomatic status of bipolar II disorder. *Arch Gen Psychiatry* 2003;60:261–9.

26. Freeman MP, Smith KW, Freeman SA et al. The impact of reproductive events on the course of bipolar disorder in women. *J Clin Psychiatry* 2002;63:284–7.

27. Koukopoulos A, Sani G, Koukopoulos AE et al. Duration and stability of the rapid-cycling course: a long-term personal follow-up of 109 patients. *J Affect Disord* 2003;73:75–85.

28. Almeida OP, Fenner S. Bipolar disorder: similarities and differences between patients with illness onset before and after 65 years of age. *Int Psychogeriatr* 2002;14:311–22.

29. Calabrese JR, Hirschfeld RM, Reed M et al. Impact of bipolar disorder on a US community sample. *J Clin Psychiatry* 2003;64:425–32.

30. Rhee SH, Hewitt JK, Corley RP, Stallings MC. The validity of analyses testing the etiology of comorbidity between two disorders: a review of family studies. *J Child Psychol Psychiatry* 2003;44:612–36.

31. Frank E, Cyranowski JM, Rucci P et al. Clinical significance of lifetime panic spectrum symptoms in the treatment of patients with bipolar I disorder. *Arch Gen Psychiatry* 2002;59:905–11.

32. Dalton EJ, Cate-Carter TD, Mundo E et al. Suicide risk in bipolar patients: the role of co-morbid substance use disorders. *Bipolar Disord* 2003;5:58–61.

33. Angst F, Stassen HH, Clayton PJ, Angst J. Mortality of patients with mood disorders: follow-up over 34–38 years. *J Affect Disord* 2002;68:167–81.

Cannabis and psychosis

Zerrin Atakan FRCPsych
National Psychosis Unit, Bethlem Royal Hospital, Beckenham, Kent, UK

Cannabis has been known to mankind since the third millennium BC. It is the most widely used psychoactive substance, and is significantly more likely to be used by people with psychotic disorders than by individuals in the general population. Interestingly, it was being used 150 years ago to treat 'insanity', while also being recognized as increasing the risk of 'madness', especially among young persons.[1]

Over the past few years there has been a revival of interest in the links between cannabis and psychosis. The reported range of lifetime cannabis use varies from 8% to 86% in individuals with psychosis.[2] Such a high level of comorbidity raises questions about the etiology, progress and outcome of the psychotic illness.

Biochemistry of cannabis

Cannabis is a complex plant containing over 400 chemical elements and 60 compounds. Two of the major compounds are tetrahydrocannabinol (Δ-9-THC) and cannabidiol (CBD).

Δ-9-THC, the psychoactive ingredient, is thought to precipitate psychosis in vulnerable individuals and to trigger a relapse of symptoms among psychotic patients.[3] Cannabinoid receptors are co-localized with the dopaminergic system in the brain and Δ-9-THC increases the release of dopamine.[4] This may explain the worsening of psychotic symptoms with acute intoxication.

CBD is devoid of the typical psychological effects associated with Δ-9-THC, but has anti-anxiety and possibly antipsychotic effects in humans.[5,6] In animal studies, it appears to have a profile similar to atypical neuroleptics.[6] One of the reasons why patients with psychosis use cannabis may be to achieve relief of tension via the anti-anxiety effect of CBD. However, the Δ-9-THC component of cannabis will increase the risk of exacerbation of psychotic symptoms. Some street cannabis (i.e. skunk) is known to have very high levels of Δ-9-THC but low levels of CBD.

In the strict scientific sense, it is incorrect to use the term 'cannabis' when the plant itself contains compounds that have a variety of different pharmacological effects. However, for ease of reference, this article uses the word 'cannabis' synonymously with 'Δ-9-THC'.

Long-term effects of cannabis on cognition

There are mixed views about the long-term effects of cannabis on cognitive function. A recent multicenter study found that long-term cannabis users performed significantly poorer in tests of verbal memory and attention, compared with short-term users and a control group; the tests were conducted when the cannabis users were not suffering the effects of acute Δ-9-THC intoxication.[7] However, the majority of studies have provided no evidence of cognitive impairment in chronic cannabis users, compared with matched healthy control subjects, based on performance in a range of neuropsychological tasks undertaken after abstinence from cannabis use for more than 24 hours.[8] Individuals with psychotic disorders who show mild-to-moderate abuse of substances, in particular alcohol and cannabis, do not exhibit more cognitive impairment than those who do not use the substances.[9]

Cannabis and dependence

Previously, it was thought that cannabis use did not cause dependence, tolerance or withdrawal symptoms, but more recent evidence disproves these views.[3,10] The results of a 21-year longitudinal study examining cannabis dependence and psychotic symptoms among young people show that development of dependence is associated with increased rates of psychotic symptoms, even after pre-existing symptoms and other factors are taken into account.[11] Similar dependence characteristics were observed in a recent study of prisoners.[12]

The link between cannabis and psychosis

Whilst the use of cannabis has been increasing steeply in many countries, the age of initial use has been decreasing.[3,13] With relaxation of the law and wide availability of the drug in many countries, cannabis use is becoming more common than cigarette smoking, especially with the growing disapproval of tobacco use among young people.[14]

The association between cannabis use in young people and subsequent risk of developing a psychotic illness has significant implications. The first major research undertaken in this area was the Swedish conscript study, involving over 50 000 subjects, which found that there was a sixfold increase in the risk of later schizophrenia among those who were heavy cannabis users at age 18 years.[15] This study was subsequently criticized for its methodology.

More recently, Zammit and colleagues re-evaluated the data from this study to take into account the criticisms and have shown that the findings are still consistent with a causal relationship.[16] However, the Swedish study does not establish whether early use is the cause of increased risk of schizophrenia or the consequence of pre-existing psychotic symptoms.

The Dunedin study is the first prospective longitudinal study of adolescent cannabis use as a risk factor for adult schizophreniform disorder, taking into account childhood psychotic symptoms antedating cannabis use.[17] A birth cohort of 1037 individuals has been followed up until the age of 26 years. As well as supporting a causal link, this study provides evidence that:
- cannabis use is not secondary to a pre-existing psychosis
- cannabis use before the age of 18 years carries a greater risk for schizophrenia than does later use
- the risk is specific to cannabis use, as opposed to use of other drugs.

Highlights in cannabis and psychosis 2003–04

WHAT'S IN?

- People with psychosis use cannabis more than the general population
- Regular cannabis use can lead to tolerance and withdrawal symptoms
- Cannabis use among young people (below the age of 18 years) increases the risk of developing psychosis approximately twofold, especially in those who have a pre-existing vulnerability
- Cannabis (Δ-9-THC) exacerbates psychotic symptoms
- Cannabis (Δ-9-THC) leads to a worse outcome, including increased hospitalization in those who are already psychotic
- Cannabis (Δ-9-THC) may increase risk of violence

WHAT'S OUT?

- Cannabis does not cause dependence
- Cannabis is a safe substance for people with psychoses and neuroses

WHAT'S UNRESOLVED?

- The biological causal link between cannabis and development of psychosis
- The long-term effect of cannabis on cognition

WHAT'S EMERGING?

- Cannabidiol being developed as an antipsychotic and anti-anxiety agent
- The study of the cannabinoid system, its agonists, antagonists and the different compounds of the plant, leading to new discoveries about the way the brain functions and the development of new medicines
- The search for specific vulnerability genes responsible for the psychogenic effects of cannabis

Another recent longitudinal study that involved a population survey examining the relationship between cannabis use and psychosis has been carried out by von Os et al.[18] Their 3-year follow-up of over 4000 individuals shows that cannabis use increases the risk of both the incidence of psychosis in previously non-psychotic individuals and a poor prognosis in those with psychotic disorder.

In contrast, Degenhardt et al. did not find any evidence of a causal link between cannabis use and the incidence of schizophrenia in their study modeling the lifespan use of cannabis in eight birth cohorts.[13] However, they and others have reported that cannabis use may precipitate disorders in those who are vulnerable to developing psychosis, and worsen the course of illness in patients who have already developed such a disorder.[13,19–21]

Phillips and colleagues studied an ultra-high-risk group and reported that cannabis use may not play an integral role in the development of psychosis in this subset. However, they concluded that cannabis use should still be considered as a candidate risk factor.[2]

As well as affecting the outcome and leading to exacerbation of symptoms, cannabis use among patients with psychosis can also lead to behavioral disturbances, such as increased risk of violence and criminal activity.[22]

Verdoux et al. studied a non-clinical sample to investigate the interaction between cannabis use and vulnerability to psychosis. They reported that there was a positive relationship between the pre-existing level of vulnerability for psychosis and the acute effects of cannabis. Compared with individuals with low vulnerability, those with high vulnerability for psychosis were more likely to report unusual perceptions, as well as feelings of thought influence. They were also less likely to experience enhanced feelings of pleasure associated with cannabis use. The authors concluded that the public health impact of the widespread use of cannabis is considerable.[23]

It is possible that vulnerability to psychosis is mediated through sensitivity to environmental risk factors, such as being reared by dysfunctional families, paternal absence, maternal cannabis use, birth complications and adverse life events.[24] In support of this view, a recent study examining the distribution of cannabinoid receptors in fetal brain showed intense expression of these receptors in the hippocampus and amygdala.[25] The authors postulate that this finding indicates that these limbic structures might be particularly vulnerable to prenatal cannabis exposure.

Particular races, as well as particular individuals, may also be genetically more vulnerable than others to the effects of cannabis in developing psychosis. Further research is required to examine possible genotype–environment interactions.

References

1. Mills JH. *Cannabis Britannica*. Oxford: Oxford University Press, 2003.

2. Phillips LJ, Curry C, Yung AR et al. Cannabis use is not associated with the development of psychosis in an 'ultra' high-risk group. *Aus N Z J Psych* 2002;36:800–806.

3. Johns A. Psychiatric effects of cannabis. *Br J Psychiatry* 2001;178: 116–22.

4. Fritzsche M. Impaired information processing triggers altered states of consciousness. *Med Hypotheses* 2002;58:352–8.

5. Zuardi AW, Morais SL, Guimaraes FS, Mechoulam R. Anti-psychotic effect of cannabidiol. *J Clin Psychiatry* 1995;56:485–6.

6. Zuardi AW, Guimaraes FS. Cannabidiol as an anxiolytic and antipsychotic. In: Mathre ML, ed. *Cannabis in Medical Practice*. Jefferson, NC, USA: McFarland & Company, 1997.

7. Solowij N, Stephens RS, Roffman RA et al. Cognitive functioning of long-term heavy cannabis users seeking treatment. *JAMA* 2002;287:1123–31.

8. Pope HG Jr. Cannabis, cognition and confounding. *JAMA* 2002; 287:1172–4.

9. Pencer A, Addington J. Substance use and cognition in early psychosis. *J Psychiatry Neurosci* 2003;28: 48–54.

10. Haney M, Ward AS et al. Abstinence symptoms following smoked marijuana in humans. *Psychopharmacology* 1999;141: 395–404.

11. Fergusson DM, Horwood LJ, Swain-Campbell NR. Cannabis dependence and psychotic symptoms in young people. *Psychol Med* 2003;33:15–21.

12. Farrell M, Boys A, Bebbington P et al. Psychosis and drug dependence: results from a national survey of prisoners. *Br J Psychiatry* 2002;181: 393–8.

13. Degenhardt L, Hall W, Lynskey M. Testing hypotheses about the relationship between cannabis use and psychosis. *Drug Alcohol Depend* 2003;71:37–48.

14. Rey JM, Tennant CC. Cannabis and mental health. *BMJ* 2002;325: 1183–4.

15. Andreasson S, Allebeck P, Engstrom A, Rydberg U. Cannabis and schizophrenia. A longitudinal study of Swedish conscripts. *Lancet* 1987;2:1483–6.

16. Zammit S, Allebeck P, Andreasson S et al. Self reported cannabis use as a risk factor for schizophrenia in Swedish conscripts of 1969: historical cohort study. *BMJ* 2002;325:1199–1201.

17. Arseneault L, Cannon M, Poulton R et al. Cannabis use in adolescence and risk for adult psychosis: longitudinal prospective study. *BMJ* 2002;325:1212–13.

18. van Os J, Bak M, Hanssen M et al. Cannabis use and psychosis: a longitudinal population-based study. *Am J Epidemiol* 2002;156:319–27.

19. Degenhardt L, Hall W. Cannabis and psychosis. *Curr Psychiatry Rep* 2002;4:191–6.

20. Degenhardt L. The link between cannabis use and psychosis: furthering the debate. *Psychol Med* 2003;33:3–6.

21. Mueser KT, Yarnold PR, Rosenberg SD et al. Substance use disorder in hospitalized severely mentally ill psychiatric patients: prevalence, correlates and subgroups. *Schizophr Bull* 2000;26:179–92.

22. Miles H, Johnson S, Amponsah-Afuwape S et al. Characteristics of subgroups of individuals with psychotic illness and a comorbid substance use disorder. *Pscyhiatr Serv* 2003;54:554–61.

23. Verdoux H, Gindre C, Sorbara F et al. Effects of cannabis and psychosis vulnerability in daily life: an experience sampling test study. *Psychol Med* 2003;33:23–32.

24. van Os J, Verdoux H. Environmental and psychosocial aspects of genetic research psychiatry. *Encephale* 1998;24:125–31.

25. Wang X, Dow-Edwards D, Keller E, Hurd YL. Preferential limbic expression of the cannabinoid receptor mRNA in the human fetal brain. *Neuroscience* 2003; 118:681–94.

Non-pharmacological treatments for anxiety disorders

Jean Cottraux MD PhD
Anxiety Disorder Unit, Hôpital Neurologique, Lyon, France

Cognitive–behavioral therapy (CBT) has been demonstrated to be effective in all the categories of anxiety disorders defined in DSM-IV. There is no strong evidence that other non-drug treatments, such as psychodynamic therapy, supportive therapy or neurosurgery, are effective.[1]

This chapter focuses on recent research in four major categories of anxiety disorders: post-traumatic stress disorder (PTSD), social phobia, specific phobias and generalized anxiety disorder (GAD).

Post-traumatic stress disorder

It is now possible to evaluate the two main tools that have been proposed for the treatment of PTSD: CBT and psychological debriefing.

Cognitive–behavioral therapy. Van Etten and Taylor conducted a meta-analysis of 61 treatment outcome studies for adult patients with PTSD, which made various comparisons between pharmacological therapies, psychological therapies (CBT, eye movement desensitization reprocessing [EMDR], relaxation training, hypnotherapy and psychodynamic therapy) and control conditions (pill placebo, waiting-list controls, supportive psychotherapies and non-saccadic EMDR control).[2] Psychological therapies were found to have significantly lower dropout rates than pharmacological treatments (14% versus 32%). This attrition rate was uniformly low. Follow-up results were available only for CBT and EMDR; outcome was maintained at 15-week follow-up. The main finding of this meta-analysis was that, in terms of PTSD symptom reduction, psychological therapies were more effective than drug therapies and both were more effective than controls.

Using CBT as a benchmark, another meta-analysis found that EMDR was no more effective than other exposure techniques. Moreover, dismantling EMDR into its components showed that saccadic ocular movements were not crucial to improvement in PTSD patients. No incremental effects due to eye movements were found when EMDR was compared with a package including all its components except for saccadic eye movements. Hence, EMDR is merely one of the numerous ways of presenting the well-established CBT methods of exposure in imagination to feared situations and restructuring of the cognitive schemas related to excessive appraisal of danger.[3]

Debriefing for PTSD prevention. Psychological debriefing was introduced as an early, short-term, single intervention that takes place in the immediate aftermath of the trauma (within 48 hours). This approach has been strongly advocated and widely used in many countries, but well-designed evaluative studies have reported negative outcomes following debriefing.

A meta-analysis of 11 high-quality randomized controlled trials has recently reported that single-session debriefing does not reduce distress, depression or anxiety, nor does it prevent PTSD.[4] Moreover, in one important trial, included in this meta-analysis, the risk of developing PTSD has been found to be higher in patients who receive debriefing than in those who do not. The authors therefore concluded that compulsory debriefing should cease. It appears that debriefing sensitizes patients, instead of enhancing the habituation process. However, controversy over the effects of debriefing is still heated.[5]

Cognitive therapy, pharmacology or exposure for social phobia?

A meta-analysis of 42 treatment-outcome trials has shown that exposure alone, pure cognitive therapy alone or social skills training alone are no more effective than placebo in treating social phobia.

> **Highlights in non-pharmacological treatment of anxiety disorders** *2003–04*
>
> **WHAT'S IN?**
> - Virtual reality for flying phobias
> - Cognitive–behavioral therapy for post-traumatic stress disorder
> - Cognitive–behavioral therapy for social phobia
> - Cognitive–behavioral therapy for generalized anxiety disorder in older adults
>
> **WHAT'S OUT?**
> - Systematic desensitization for flying phobia
> - Debriefing for preventing post-traumatic stress disorder
> - Eye movement as an explanation for eye movement desensitization and reprocessing effects

However, there is a significant positive effect when a combination of cognitive therapy and exposure is used.[6]

In contrast, a more recent trial has reported positive effects with exposure alone. Over 300 patients with social phobia were randomized to receive the selective serotonin-reuptake inhibitor, sertraline, or placebo for 24 weeks, with or without the addition of exposure therapy. The initial analysis found that sertraline alone and exposure plus sertraline were significantly superior to placebo. At 1-year follow-up (28 weeks after the end of the treatment period), psychometric test scores were compared with results immediately after the treatment period. Patients receiving exposure therapy alone showed a further improvement which was statistically significant ($p < 0.01$). Patients in the placebo group also showed a further improvement which was significant, though at a lesser level ($p < 0.05$). By contrast, sertraline given alone or in combination with exposure therapy showed a tendency towards deterioration after the completion of treatment when compared with placebo or exposure alone at week 52.

The results of this study are in line with most studies reporting on patients' progress after cessation of drug treatment or CBT in anxiety disorders or depression. However, in this study the placebo group also demonstrated some improvement.

Virtual reality for specific phobias

A controlled study of low statistical power introduced virtual reality as a tool to expose patients with acrophobia to feared stimuli, and reported positive results.[8] A subsequent controlled trial involving 20 subjects who were phobic about flying found that treatment using virtual reality was superior to being placed on a waiting list.[9]

More recently, Wiederhold et al. have conducted a trial to compare the effectiveness of virtual reality graded exposure with imagined exposure.[10] They randomly assigned 30 participants with a DSM-IV diagnosis of specific phobia about flying to one of three groups: virtual reality with no physiological feedback; virtual reality with physiological feedback; or systematic desensitization with imagined exposure therapy. Sessions were carried out once a week for 8 weeks. Only 10% of the patients receiving systematic desensitization with imagined exposure were able to fly without medication or alcohol at 3-month post-treatment follow-up, compared with 80% of those receiving virtual reality sessions with no physiological feedback and 100% of patients receiving virtual reality sessions with physiological feedback.[10]

Less positive outcomes have been reported by Maltby et al.[11] Forty-five participants who refused to fly during a screening test and who also met the DSM-IV criteria for specific phobia, agoraphobia or panic disorder with agoraphobia were randomly assigned to five sessions of either virtual reality exposure or attention-placebo group treatment. Post-treatment, 65% of participants in the virtual reality group flew during a test flight, compared with 57% of participants in the attention-placebo group; this difference was not significant. Results of a standardized self-assessment measure of flight anxiety showed significant improvement in both treatment groups in this study, but the virtual reality group showed a statistically significant outcome in four of the five domains. At 6-month follow-up, most between-group differences had vanished but the virtual reality group still reported a statistically significant improvement in outcome in one domain.

Treatment of generalized anxiety disorder in older adults

In a study by Wetherell et al., 75 older adults (mean age 67 years) with GAD were randomly assigned to CBT, a discussion group organized around worry-provoking topics, or a waiting period. Participants in both active treatment groups improved relative to the waiting list group. Although CBT participants improved on more measures than the discussion group, the difference between these two groups was significant only immediately after treatment and not at 6-month follow-up. The results show that brief treatment of late-life GAD is beneficial, but do not establish that CBT is superior to discussion group intervention.

Another recent trial involving GAD patients compared CBT with a minimal contact control group. Eighty-five adults with GAD, aged 60 years or older, were assessed for worry, anxiety, depression, specific fears and quality of life. Results of both completer and intent-to-treat analyses revealed significant improvement in worry, anxiety, depression and quality of life favoring CBT over the minimal contact group. Of the patients receiving CBT, 45% were classified as responders, compared with only 8% in the minimal contact group. The gains for patients in the CBT group were maintained or enhanced over a 1-year follow-up. However, the post-treatment scores for patients receiving CBT did not indicate a return to normal functioning.

More research and meta-analyses are needed to resolve the debate on whether better outcomes are achieved with specific or non-specific psychological interventions for GAD.

References

1. Cottraux J. Non-pharmacological treatments for anxiety disorders. *Dialogues Clin Neurosci* 2002;4: 305–19.

2. Van Etten ML, Taylor S. Comparative efficacy of treatments for post-traumatic stress disorder: a meta-analysis. *Clin Psychol Psychother* 1998;5:126–44.

3. Davidson PR, Parker KCH. Eye movement desensitization and reprocessing (EMDR): a meta analysis. *J Consult Clin Psychol* 2001;69:305–16.

4. Rose S, Bisson J, Wessely S. *Psychological debriefing for preventing post-traumatic stress disorder (PTSD)*. The Cochrane Library, Issue 4, 2003. Oxford: Update Software Ltd.

5. Wessely S, Deahl M. Psychological debriefing is a waste of time. *Br J Psychiatry* 2003;183:12–14.

6. Fedoroff IC, Taylor S. Psychological and pharmacological treatments of social phobia: a meta-analysis. *J Clin Psychopharmacol* 2001;21:311–24.

7. Haug TT, Blomhoff S, Hellstrom K et al. Exposure therapy and sertraline in social phobia: 1-year follow-up of a randomised controlled trial. *Br J Psychiatry* 2003;182:312–18.

8. Rothbaum BO, Hodges LF, Kooper R et al. Effectiveness of computer-generated (virtual reality) graded exposure in the treatment of acrophobia. *Am J Psychiatry* 1995;152:626–8.

9. Muhlberger A, Herrmann MJ, Wiedemann GC, Ellgring H, Pauli P. Repeated exposure of flight phobics to flights in virtual reality. *Behav Res Ther* 2001;39:1033–50.

10. Wiederhold BK, Jang DP, Gevirtz RG et al. The treatment of fear of flying: a controlled study of imaginal and virtual reality graded exposure therapy. *IEEE Trans Inf Technol Biomed* 2002;6:218–23.

11. Maltby N, Kirsch J, Mayers M, Allen GJ. Virtual reality exposure therapy for the treatment of fear of flying: a controlled investigation. *J Consult Clin Psychol* 2002;70: 1112–18.

12. Wetherell JL, Gatz M, Craske MG. Treatment of generalized anxiety disorder in older adults. *J Consult Clin Psychol* 2003;71: 31–40.

13. Stanley MA, Beck JG, Novy DM et al. Cognitive–behavioral treatment of late-life generalized anxiety disorder. *J Consult Clin Psychol* 2003;71:309–12.

Drug treatment of generalized anxiety disorder

Malcolm Lader OBE DSc PhD MD FRCPsych FMedSci
Institute of Psychiatry, King's College London, UK

Anxiety is a very common symptom that accompanies stress, physical illnesses and adverse events in everyday life. The most well-defined form of anxiety is termed generalized anxiety disorder (GAD), which is the most prevalent of the group of mental illnesses called the anxiety disorders. It is usually treated by primary care physicians; only the most severe, persistent and disabling cases are referred to psychiatrists.

The diagnostic criteria for GAD, as defined by ICD-10,[1] are listed in Table 1. GAD comprises a sense of apprehensive expectation accompanied by a range of physical symptoms, including sweating, palpitations and muscle tension. GAD is a chronic fluctuating or relapsing disorder, which affects men and women in about equal proportions. It has a peak age of onset in the 20s and a peak in the number of presentations for treatment in the 30s. GAD is commonly comorbid with other anxiety disorders and depression.

General management
General assessment should include family history (GAD is often familial), personality traits, attitudes to symptoms, the physical symptom pattern, expectations of treatment, and willingness to accept drug and non-drug treatments. In all but the most severe cases, the first line of treatment should be psychological, ranging from simple directive counseling to cognitive–behavioral treatment (see page 37).[2]

Pharmacotherapy
The involvement of the inhibitory neurotransmitter, γ-aminobutyric acid (GABA), in the underlying mechanisms of anxiety has long

> **TABLE 1**
>
> **ICD-10 criteria for generalized anxiety disorder**
>
> The essential feature is anxiety, which is generalized and persistent but not restricted to, or even strongly predominating in, any particular environmental circumstances (i.e. it is 'free-floating'). As in other anxiety disorders, the dominant symptoms are highly variable, but complaints of continuous feelings of nervousness, trembling, muscular tension, sweating, lightheadedness, palpitations, dizziness and epigastric discomfort are common. Fears that the sufferer or a relative will shortly become ill or have an accident are often expressed, together with a variety of other worries and forebodings. This disorder is more common in women and is often related to chronic environmental stress. Its course is variable but tends to be fluctuating and chronic
>
> **Diagnostic guidelines**
>
> The patient must have primary symptoms of anxiety on most days for at least several weeks at a time, and usually for several months. These symptoms should usually involve elements of:
>
> - apprehension (e.g. worries about future misfortunes, feeling 'on edge', difficulty in concentrating)
> - motor tension (e.g. restless fidgeting, tension headaches, trembling, inability to relax)
> - autonomic overactivity (e.g. lightheadedness, sweating, tachycardia or tachypnea, epigastric discomfort, dizziness, dry mouth)

been assumed.[3] This assumption is based on the effectiveness of the benzodiazepines in assuaging anxiety, as they potentiate GABA. Some commonly prescribed anxiolytic benzodiazepines are listed in Table 2. In many countries, diazepam remains the most popular agent. Some benzodiazepines are long-acting and are therefore appropriate for maintaining a smooth background level of anxiolysis; others are shorter-acting and more appropriate for combating fluctuating levels of anxiety. The therapeutic effects of benzodiazepines are too well-known to need repetition.[4] Their effects are not specifically anti-anxiety but more generally anti-arousal, with sedation and reduction of hypervigilance – and also lowering of other emotions, even positive ones such as pleasure.

TABLE 2

Some drug treatments for generalized anxiety disorder (note that doses may vary from licensed doses in depression)

	Usual dose (mg/day)	Unwanted effects
Benzodiazepines		
Long-acting		
Diazepam	10–30	Sedation
Chlordiazepoxide	10–40	Drowsiness
Intermediate-acting		
Lorazepam	1–6	Sedation, dizziness
Alprazolam	0.25–4	Drowsiness, withdrawal
Clonazepam	0.25–4	Fatigue
Antidepressants		
Tricyclic antidepressants		
Imipramine	75–225	Sedation, dry mouth
Clomipramine	25–150	Sedation, weight gain
Selective serotonin-reuptake inhibitors		
Fluoxetine	10–40	Nausea, insomnia
Paroxetine	10–40	Nausea, withdrawal
Sertraline	50–200	Nausea, insomnia
Citalopram	10–40	Nausea, dry mouth
Serotonin–norepinephrine-reuptake inhibitor		
Venlafaxine	37.5–150	Nausea, dizziness
Other medications		
Buspirone	15–45	Dizziness, nausea
Propranolol	45–120	Sedation, depression

In addition, muscle relaxation is induced. Somatic symptoms are reduced, perhaps more than psychological symptoms. Long-term efficacy has not been established.[5]

The general sedation caused by benzodiazepines also leads to impairment of psychological performance, which can be quite marked, particularly when the drug is taken in combination with alcohol. Reaction times are prolonged and muscular activity becomes uncoordinated, hence driving ability may be seriously compromised. Occasionally, there is a release of emotions (e.g. aggression) – the so-called paradoxical effect.[6]

The popularity of benzodiazepines has waned in many countries over the past 10–15 years because of these adverse effects, but also because of an increasing awareness of withdrawal and dependence problems.[7] These problems range from a mild rebound of anxiety to a major, prolonged and disabling syndrome (Table 3). Patients with a history of substance or alcohol abuse are particularly likely to experience symptoms.

As well as discontinuation problems, addicts commonly abuse benzodiazepines, taken alone orally, snorted or injected, or in conjunction with heroin and cocaine.

Antidepressants

It has become increasingly apparent that serotonin (5-hydroxytryptamine, 5-HT) is a crucial neurotransmitter in the mediation of emotions. Indeed, the inhibitory effects

TABLE 3

Symptoms of withdrawal from benzodiazepines

Psychological

- Apprehension
- Irritability
- Insomnia
- Dysphoria

Physiological

- Tremor
- Muscle spasms
- Loss of appetite and weight
- Malaise

Perceptual disturbances

- Hypersensitivity to light, sound and touch
- Feelings of motion
- Depersonalization

Highlights in drug treatment of generalized anxiety disorder 2003–04

WHAT'S IN?

- Selective serotonin-reuptake inhibitors (SSRIs) becoming the drugs of choice
- Venlafaxine also effective – used as second-line agent
- Long-term drug treatment combined with cognitive–behavioral treatment
- Tapering of all medications, typically over 1–4 weeks

WHAT'S OUT?

- Use of benzodiazepines – except as short-term adjuncts
- Use of antihistamines, antipsychotics, β-blockers
- Drug treatment of minor anxiety conditions
- Drug treatment of the 'worried well'

WHAT'S NEEDED?

- Long-term trials of SSRIs, selective norepinephrine-reuptake inhibitors and putative new anxiolytics
- Studies of optimal combinations of drug and non-drug treatments
- Studies of compliance/adherence to drug treatment including how to improve it

of GABA in lessening anxiety may be focused on serotonin pathways in the limbic system of the brain.

Whatever the mechanism, numerous studies have shown the efficacy of tricyclic antidepressants and, more recently, the selective serotonin-reuptake inhibitors (SSRIs) as anti-anxiety agents.[8,9] Another effective compound is the non-selective reuptake inhibitor, venlafaxine.[10] Currently, the SSRIs or venlafaxine are the preferred anxiolytics, because the tricyclics have a much less favorable adverse event profile.

The anxiolytic effect of SSRIs and venlafaxine differs from that of benzodiazepines in typically being delayed for at least 1 week, and occasionally for several weeks. Moreover, some patients experience a short-lived upsurge in anxiety with some of these drugs, and even the onset of panic. Many prescribers therefore start with a low dose and increase it only if the drug is well-tolerated. Patients must be warned of the possibility of temporary worsening of their symptoms.

Psychic symptoms are usually helped more than physical symptoms, but the overall therapeutic effects of SSRIs and venlafaxine can be impressive. These effects usually persist as long as medication is continued. This gives a window of opportunity for psychological treatments to be applied.

Adverse effects are the same as those noted when the drugs are used to treat depression. Discontinuation can give rise to some evanescent symptoms, particularly in the case of paroxetine and venlafaxine, but these are usually mild. Abuse does not occur.

Azapirones

Buspirone is available as an anxiolytic.[11] It acts on the serotonin system. It has more effect on psychological than physical symptoms, and is delayed in its onset of action. Buspirone does not induce dependence.

Other drugs

Antihistamines are generally sedative. They can reduce anxiety, but usually also induce drowsiness.[12] Anticholinergic side effects may also supervene.

Low doses of antipsychotic drugs have been used as anxiolytics, but should be avoided because of the risk of extrapyramidal side effects, such as tardive dyskinesia.[13]

β-adrenoreceptor antagonists (β-blockers) may help some patients with anxiety who have physical symptoms such as palpitations and tremor.[14] They are traditionally used to treat situational anxiety, such as stage-fright.

Drugs in development

Several novel leads are being pursued as potential new treatments for various anxiety disorders. These promising approaches include corticotropin-releasing factor antagonists (CRF_1 antagonists), substance P antagonists (NK_1 antagonists), and compounds related chemically to GABA (such as gaboxadol and pregabalin).

Treatment strategies

Each treatment plan must be tailored to the individual patient, taking into consideration his or her attitudes to drugs and psychological therapy, expectations of response and side effects, and symptom pattern.

Medication should be regarded as a temporary expedient, giving symptom relief while more general management strategies are instituted. The severity of the symptoms and the associated impairments – interpersonal, social and occupational – need careful assessment to ensure that drugs are not being prescribed unnecessarily.

In a nutshell, modern anti-anxiety drug treatment concentrates on the careful administration of adequate doses of an SSRI. Venlafaxine is less well-tolerated, and many experts hold it in reserve. If immediate symptom relief is imperative, it may be appropriate to prescribe a benzodiazepine for up to 4 weeks in total, in conjunction with the SSRI. The dose of the benzodiazepine should be halved during the final week.

References

1. World Health Organization. *International Statistical Classification of Diseases and Related Health Problems – 10th revision.* Geneva: World Health Organization, 1992.

2. Gould RA, Otto MW, Pollack MH et al. Cognitive behavioural and pharmacological treatment of generalised anxiety disorder: a preliminary meta-analysis. *Behav Ther* 1997;28:285–305.

3. Davidson JR. Pharmacology of generalised anxiety disorder. *J Clin Psych* 2001;62(suppl 11):46–50.

4. Ashton H. Guidelines for the rational use of benzodiazepines: when and what to use. *Drugs* 1994;48: 25–40.

5. Schweitzer E, Rickels K. Pharmacological treatment of generalised anxiety disorder. In: Mavissakalian MR, Prien RF, eds. *Long-Term Treatments of Anxiety Disorders.* Washington DC: American Psychiatric Press, 1996: 201–20.

6. Rosenbaum JF, Woods SW, Groves JE et al. Emergence of hostility during alprazolam treatment. *Am J Psychiatry* 1984;141:792–3.

7. Lader M. Benzodiazepines. A risk-benefit profile. *CNS Drugs* 1994;1: 377–87.

8. Rocca P, Fonzo V, Scotta M et al. Paroxetine efficacy in the treatment of generalised anxiety disorder. *Acta Psychiatr Scand* 1997;95:444–50.

9. Gorman JM, Kent JM. SSRIs and SNRIs: broad spectrum of efficacy beyond major depression. *J Clin Psychiatry* 1999;60(suppl 4):33–8.

10. Rickels K, Pollack MH, Sheehan DV et al. Efficacy of extended release venlafaxine in nondepressed outpatients with generalised anxiety disorder. *Am J Psychiatry* 2000;157: 968–74.

11. Sussman N. Treatment of anxiety with buspirone. *Psychiatr Ann* 1987;17:114–20.

12. Ferreri M, Hantouche EG. Recent clinical trials of hydroxyzine in generalised anxiety disorder. *Acta Psychiatr Scand Suppl* 1998;393: 102–8.

13. Chou JCY, Sussman N. Neuroleptics in anxiety. *Psychiatr Ann* 1988;18:172–5.

14. Hayes PE, Schulz SC. Beta-blockers in anxiety disorders. *J Affect Disord* 1987;13:119–30.

Recurrent brief depression

David Baldwin FRCPsych

Clinical Neurosciences Research Division, Faculty of Medicine, Health and Life Sciences, University of Southampton, UK

Recurrent brief depression (RBD) has a long history. In 1921, Kraepelin included short and mild depressive states within the overall category of manic-depressive illness.[1] Eight years later, Paskind noted that patients with brief but recurring depressions were common in primary care, and an association with suicidal behavior was noted by Buzzard et al. shortly thereafter.[2,3] Despite this, RDB has appeared in official classification schemes only in the past decade, being listed within depressive disorders in the ICD-10 and with 'disorders worthy of further investigation' in the DSM-IV.

The groundbreaking prospective epidemiological study led by Angst ('the Zurich study') indicates that RBD has a lifetime prevalence of approximately 10%, similar to that of major depression. Other community and primary care studies suggest a point prevalence of 2–7%. Although apparently common, RBD has not been researched extensively: a computerized literature search conducted through PubMed in December 2003 identified only 20 papers published in the period 2002–03.

Common and comorbid

Two recent community studies support the contention that RBD is a common and disabling condition.[4,5] In a Sardinian mixed urban and rural community sample (n = 1040), the overall lifetime prevalence was estimated to be 7.6% (5.8% in men, 9.0% in women). The disorder was found to be most common in younger adults.[4]

A lower lifetime prevalence (2.6%) is suggested by the findings of the prospective Early Developmental Stages of Psychopathology Study performed in young adults (aged 14–24 years at baseline) living in Munich (n = 3021).[5]

There are still no data available on the point and lifetime prevalence of RBD in secondary care samples.[6]

Data from the Zurich study suggest that RBD and major depression are similar in terms of age of onset, family history, social class, presentation for treatment and physical comorbidity.[7] The results of the Munich study indicate that RBD shows less comorbidity with panic disorder, social phobia, generalized anxiety disorder and obsessive–compulsive disorder, and more comorbidity with post-traumatic stress disorder, than does major depression.[5] The Sardinian study reveals significantly greater comorbidity with dysthymia, social phobia, panic disorder and substance abuse in subjects with RBD than in the overall study sample.[4]

Association with suicidal behavior

The Zurich study found that RBD is associated with a fourfold increase in the risk of attempted suicide.[7] In the Munich sample, suicide attempts were reported by 7.8% of subjects with RBD and 11.9% with major depression, but by no subjects with 'combined depression' (RBD plus major depression);[6] this last finding is in sharp contrast to earlier observations in clinical samples. The association of RBD with suicide attempts was also seen in the Sardinian sample, but only in those with combined depression.[4] Small study numbers probably account for these disparate findings.

Attempts to elucidate the pathophysiology

Few attempts have been made to identify the pathophysiology of RBD. As well as showing substantial longitudinal comorbidity with major depression, many patients with RBD fulfil diagnostic criteria for borderline personality disorder.

The results of neuroendocrine challenge tests indicate that RBD and major depression are both associated with blunting of the response to thyrotropin-releasing hormone, whereas borderline personality disorder is not. With the dexamethasone suppression test, RBD and borderline personality disorder are both associated with less abnormality than is seen in patients with major depression.[8]

Highlights in recurrent brief depression 2003–04

WHAT'S IN?

- Recognition of the need for further research in clinical samples
- Epidemiological studies of recurrent brief depression (RBD) in young adults
- Investigation of the neurobiology of RBD
- Single-case analyses and case series of open-label treatment with antidepressants

WHAT'S OUT?

- Scepticism about existence of RBD
- Proposed inclusion of RBD within the bipolar spectrum
- Idea that RBD is just a form of borderline personality disorder

The significant association of RBD with adult attention deficit hyperactivity disorder suggests that dopaminergic function might be perturbed in RBD. A lifetime diagnosis of RBD was recorded in 70% of a secondary-care sample of adults (n = 40) with attention deficit hyperactivity disorder, whereas attention deficit hyperactivity disorder had a point prevalence of 40% in psychiatric outpatients with a primary diagnosis of RBD.[9]

Are we closer to an effective treatment?

Epidemiological studies indicate that many people with RBD receive treatment, but no treatment has been proven effective in these patients. Data from the Zurich study indicate that the short-term (1-year) outcome in patients with RBD is improved with psychotropic drugs, but the long-term (8-year) outcome is similar in treated and untreated patients.[10]

Although a double-blind placebo-controlled study in patients with a history of repeated suicide attempts but without major depression (n = 107) reported that fluoxetine treatment conferred no advantage in preventing brief depressive episodes or associated deliberate self-harm,[11] results of a more recent open-label case series (n = 17) suggest that it may be beneficial in reducing the number and duration of depressive episodes.[12]

A single case analysis using before and after data suggests that the selective norepinephrine-reuptake inhibitor, reboxetine, was helpful in reducing the burden of brief depressive episodes.[13] A multicenter randomized controlled trial in patients with repeated deliberate self-harm (many of whom would probably fulfil criteria for RBD) suggests that brief cognitive therapy was no more efficacious than 'treatment as usual'.[14]

A plea for more research

Clinicians will be disappointed that there are still no proven treatments for what appears to be a common and impairing condition. However, such treatments will become available only after the psychopathological features of RBD in primary and secondary care samples have been characterized more extensively.

Investigations of the benefits and risks of intervention in patients with RBD are hard to undertake because of the substantial comorbidity and association with suicidal behavior, but the absence of an accepted treatment confirms the need for rigorous double-blind randomized placebo-controlled treatment studies.[15]

References

1. Kraepelin E. Manic depressive insanity and paranoia. In: Robertson, G (ed). *Textbook of Psychiatry.* Vols 3 and 4 (translated from 8th German edition by: Barclay M). Edinburgh: E & S Livingstone, 1921.

2. Paskind HA. Brief attacks of manic-depressive depression. *Arch Neurol Psychiatry* 1929;22:123–34.

3. Buzzard EF, Miller HE, Riddoch G et al. Discussion on the diagnosis and treatment of the milder forms of the manic-depressive psychosis. *Proc R Soc Med* 1930;23:881–95.

4. Carta MG, Altamura AC, Hardoy MC et al. Is recurrent brief depression an expression of mood disorders in young people? Results of a large community sample. *Eur Arch Psychiatry Clin Neurosci* 2003;253: 149–53.

5. Pezawas L, Wittchen H-U, Pfister H et al. Recurrent brief depressive disorder reinvestigated: a community sample of adolescents and young adults. *Psychol Med* 2003;33:407–18.

6. Baldwin DS. Recurrent brief depression – more investigations in clinical samples are now required. *Psychol Med* 2003;33:383–6.

7. Angst J, Hochstrasser B. Recurrent brief depression: the Zurich study. *J Clin Psychiatr* 1994;55(suppl): S3–9.

8. De la Fuente JM, Bobes J, Vizuete C, Mendlewicz J. Biological nature of depressive symptoms in borderline personality disorder: endocrine comparison to recurrent brief and major depression. *J Psychiatric Res* 2002;36:137–45.

9. Hesslinger B, Tebartz van Elst L, Mochan F, Ebert D. A psychopathological study into the relationship between attention deficit hyperactivity disorder in adult patients and recurrent brief depression. *Acta Psychiatr Scand* 2003;107:385–9.

10. Hasler G, Schnyder U, Klaghofer R, Angst J. Treatment of depressive disorders with and without medication – a naturalistic study. *Pharmacopsychiatry* 2002;35:235–8.

11. Montgomery DB, Roberts A, Green M et al. Lack of efficacy of fluoxetine in recurrent brief depression and suicide attempts. *Eur Arch Psychiatry Clin Neurosci* 1994,244:211–15.

12. Stamenkovic M, Blaasbichler T, Riedere F et al. Fluoxetine treatment in patients with recurrent brief depression. *Int Clin Psychopharmacol* 2001;16:221–6.

13. Pezawas L, Stamenkovic M, Aschauer N. Successful treatment of recurrent brief depression with reboxetine – a single case analysis. *Pharmacopsychiatry* 2002;35:75–6.

14. Tyrer P, Thompson S, Schmidt U et al. Randomized controlled trial of brief cognitive behaviour therapy versus treatment as usual in recurrent deliberate self-harm: the POPMACT study. *Psychol Med* 2003;33:969–76.

15. Baldwin DS, Broich K, Fritze J et al. Placebo-controlled studies in depression: necessary, ethical and feasible. *Eur Arch Psychiatry Clin Neurosci* 2003;253:22–8.

Suicide in custody

Heather Stuart PhD
Department of Community Health and Epidemiology, Queen's University, Kingston, Ontario, Canada

Suicide is the leading cause of death among adult offenders in custodial settings.[1] Inmates are up to 10 times more likely to die from suicide than their counterparts in the general population and, in many countries, the rate of inmate suicide is rising.[2]

Despite the scope of the problem, little attention has been paid to this area of research. A literature search for English-language publications indexed in ClinPsych, EMBASE, HealthSTAR and MEDLINE for the years 1992–2003 identified only 258 unique citations, accounting for 3.2% of all articles on prisons and jails, and only 0.5% of all articles on suicide. Although research is progressing slowly, the epidemiological studies that have been published recently reinforce the ubiquitous nature of inmate suicide internationally, and highlight the public health importance of suicide as the leading preventable cause of inmate death.

Scope of the problem

Custody-related deaths pose a major human rights issue as they may account for up to three-quarters of all deaths among inmates who have not yet gone to trial, and one-third of all deaths among sentenced prisoners.[1] An autopsy study of all custody-related deaths in Durban, South Africa between January 1998 and December 2000 showed that there were 102 deaths as a result of police actions (such as shootings, assaults, or assaults by police dogs) and 15 deaths among those in custody. Seven of the deaths in custody (47%) were suicides – all by hanging. In all seven cases, the deceased had been alone in a cell with access to hanging materials such as shoelaces or bed linen. Alcohol was considered to be a factor in only one of the seven cases.[3]

In 2003, two papers were published from a large epidemiological survey of psychiatric morbidity among inmates in England and Wales. The first described non-fatal suicide behavior among prisoners, and the second reviewed psychiatric morbidity and suicidality among women prisoners.[4,5] Over a quarter of male prisoners who were on remand had attempted suicide in their lifetime and one-sixth had done so in the past year. Half of the female prisoners on remand had attempted suicide in their lifetime and over a quarter had done so in the past year. In the week prior to the interview, 23% of the women prisoners had thought of suicide. Those who attempted suicide were in poorer general and mental health, and were more likely to be located in special units such as hospital wings, special handling units or segregation units.

As well as being a major cause of mortality, suicide attempts are the leading cause of inmate transfers to hospital emergency departments. The opening of a new prison allowed Scottish researchers to examine the additional workload placed on a local emergency department. During the first year of operation of the prison, 22% of the 103 emergency transfers were for treatment of deliberate self-harm, making this the leading cause of emergency medical transfers from the prison.[6]

Little is known about the frequency of suicide among young offenders. In perhaps the first study of its kind, mortality was examined in a 12-year follow-up of 3000 young offenders undergoing their first custodial sentence in Victoria, Australia in 1998–99.[7] The overall risk of death (from any cause) was nine times higher among male young offenders compared with the reference male population (15 years and under). Twenty-three suicides occurred in total (22 of these in men), comprising 24% of all deaths. Suicide in the age-matched reference population accounted for 22% of all deaths.

Suicidogenic nature of incarcerated settings
The higher frequency of suicides among those in custody who have not yet gone to trial is attributed to the initial trauma of incarceration in combination with inmate vulnerabilities, such as

mental illness, intoxication or withdrawal.[1] However, characteristics of the institution may also play a role. For example, there is typically a rapid turnover among inmates who have not yet gone to trial, which poses significant challenges for suicide prevention. These inmates may stay in custody for only a few days before being released on bail. This therefore necessitates immediate assessment procedures and makes discharge planning more challenging. Not surprisingly, the greater the absolute number of inmates being processed (i.e. the larger the jail), the less likely it is that mentally ill offenders will receive appropriate care.[8]

A qualitative study of environmental factors impacting prisoners' mental health was undertaken in a medium-security prison in a semi-rural part of southern England.[9] Prisoners identified the lack of mental stimulation, drug misuse, negative relationships with staff, bullying and a lack of family contact as some of the key mental health issues they faced. Focus groups with staff also identified aspects of the prison work environment considered relevant to inmate suicide, such as a lack of management support, negative work culture, low staff safety, high stress levels and increasing rates of staff sickness.

Psychology of inmate suicide

Two studies examined psychological factors in relation to inmate suicide. In a study of 235 consecutive admissions to a maximum-security Canadian federal prison, 17% of inmates reported a prior suicide attempt – a figure that was only slightly higher than the 13% reported by inmates in a medium-security Canadian federal prison.[10] Prisoners who survived a suicide attempt attributed their motivation to factors reflecting internal psychological pain (such as shame, guilt, fear, dread or anguish) more often than traditional psychological variables (such as hopelessness). These results may have important implications for suicide screening in correctional settings.

The second study followed prisoners through the initial phases of their remand and solitary confinement.[11] Psychological vulnerabilities were more apparent during the early phases of remand and among inmates in solitary confinement. Once prisoners

> ### Highlights in suicide in custody 2003–04
>
> #### WHAT'S IN?
> - Recognition that suicide is a major cause of death in custodial settings and in the months immediately following release
> - Integrated networks of care, including transitional planning and post-release strategies
>
> #### WHAT'S NEW?
> - Best practice guidelines for improving mental health in custodial settings and for reducing suicidality
>
> #### WHAT'S NEEDED?
> - More research on inmate suicide
> - More information on suicide in young offender populations
> - Evaluation data on the effectiveness of best practice guidelines in reducing suicidality
> - Monitoring data on the number of custodial settings that conform to best practice standards

were moved out of solitary confinement, psychological health improved. These findings are consistent with epidemiological research showing a higher-than-average suicide rate during the early phases of remand and among prisoners held in isolation cells.[1]

Best practices in suicide prevention

While it has been argued that custodial settings do not constitute the best therapeutic environment in which to treat people with mental health problems,[12] there is growing recognition that they do offer an important window of opportunity for suicide prevention – one that cannot be easily dismissed. Landmark decisions in several countries have affirmed that inmates do have the right to suicide-prevention programs and mental health care consistent with community standards.[1] Increasingly, this has come to mean systematic screening, intervention and release planning.[13]

Best practice models for inmate suicide prevention have begun to emerge. Preliminary evaluation of their effects suggests that they can reduce suicide rates even in the busiest of jail systems.[1] The most recent example of a best practice guideline focuses on community re-entry from jails for inmates with comorbid disorders – a particularly high risk group for suicide.[8] This is a comprehensive process involving four components:
- assessment of inmates' clinical and social needs, and public safety risks
- planning appropriate treatment to address these needs
- identification of community-based programs responsible for post-release planning
- coordination of the transition plan to ensure that necessary services are implemented.

By including transitional planning, this is the first guideline to make such a forceful recommendation for an integrated, system-wide approach to service delivery in correctional settings. The importance of adequate transition planning is highlighted by a report of a sevenfold increase in drug-related mortality in the first 2 weeks after release, and a fivefold increase in non-drug-related deaths in the first 12 weeks after release from prison. Suicides accounted for 10 of the 21 non-drug-related deaths in this time period.[14]

Comprehensive guidelines are important because correctional systems may not follow through with treatment once a suicide problem has been identified. In Austria, where there were 250 suicides between 1975 and 1999, the majority of cases were preceded by signs of suicidality and psychiatric problems.[2] Suicide attempts preceded half of all suicides and, in 37% of the cases, suicide threats had been reported to prison authorities. Substance abuse was identified in over half of all suicides. In one out of every five suicides, no preventive action had been implemented in spite of obvious signs of suicidality.

These results highlight the significance of suicide behaviors as precursors to suicide among inmate populations, the importance of implementing appropriate suicide screening, and the need to ensure that adequate psychiatric follow-through occurs once suicidal behaviors have been identified.[1,15]

References

1. Stuart H. Suicide behind bars. *Curr Opin Psychiatry* 2003;16:559–64.

2. Fruehwald S, Frottier P, Matschnig T, Eher R. The relevance of suicidal behaviour in jail and prison suicides. *Eur Psychiatry* 2003;18:161–5.

3. Bhana BD. Custody-related deaths in Durban, South Africa, 1998–2000. *Am J Forensic Med Pathol* 2003;24:202–7.

4. Meltzer H, Jenkins R, Singleton N et al. Non-fatal suicidal behaviour among prisoners. *Int Rev Psychiatry* 2003;15:148–9.

5. O'Brien M, Mortimer L, Singleton N, Meltzer H. Psychiatric morbidity among women prisoners in England and Wales. *Int Rev Psychiatry* 2003;15:153–7.

6. Boyce SH, Stevenson J, Jamieson IS, Campbell S. Impact of a newly opened prison on an accident and emergency department. *Emerg Med* 2003;20:48–51.

7. Coffey C, Veit F, Wolfe R et al. Mortality in young offenders: retrospective cohort study. *BMJ* 2003;326:1064–7.

8. Osher F, Steadman HJ, Barr H. A best practice approach to community reentry from jails for inmates with co-occurring disorders: The APIC Model. *Crime Delinquency* 2003;49:79–96.

9. Nurse J, Woodcock P, Ormsby J. Influence of environmental factors on mental health within prisons: focus group study. *BMJ* 2003;327:480–4.

10. Holden RR, Kroner DG. Differentiating suicidal motivations and manifestations in a forensic sample. *Can J Behav Sci* 2003;35: 35–44.

11. Anderson HS, Sestoft D, Lillebaek T et al. A longitudinal study of prisoners on remand. Repeated measures of psychopathology in the initial phase of solitary versus nonsolitary confinement. *Int J Law Psychiatry* 2003;26:165–77.

12. Daigle M. Death in our prisons (Letter to the Editor). *Can Med Assoc J* 2003;168:830.

13. Abram KM, Teplin LA, McClelland GM. Comorbidity of severe psychiatric disorders and substance use disorders among women in jail. *Am J Psychiatry* 2003;160:1007–10.

14. Bird SM, Hutchinson SJ. Male drugs-related deaths in the fortnight after release from prison: Scotland, 1996–99. *Addiction* 2003;98:185–90.

15. Wobeser WL. Death in our prisons (Letter to the Editor). *Can Med Assoc J* 2003;167:831.

Post-traumatic stress disorder after earthquakes

Metin Başoğlu MD PhD
Section of Trauma Studies, Institute of Psychiatry, Division of Psychological Medicine, King's College, London, UK

Earthquakes are common natural disasters, causing widespread destruction and casualties. The mental health hazard associated with earthquakes primarily concerns developing countries, as they suffer greater devastation and casualties from earthquakes than do industrialized nations. This is the result of the poor structural quality of buildings and lack of preparation for disasters in most developing nations. In the 20th century, 91 of the 108 major earthquakes (i.e. those with a death toll over 1000) occurred in developing countries, accounting for 76% of the 1.8 million earthquake-related deaths worldwide.[1]

Despite the extent of the problem, relatively little information is available on effective treatments for earthquake survivors. As there are no controlled studies of treatment interventions based on sound theory in adult earthquake survivors, the present review is primarily based on our own work with more than 11 000 survivors of the 1999 earthquakes in Turkey.

Mental health consequences of earthquakes

There is converging evidence that natural disasters lead to elevated rates of psychiatric morbidity.[2] Three field surveys and an epidemiological study, involving a total of 4620 survivors of the 1999 earthquakes in Turkey, have shown that post-traumatic stress disorder (PTSD) and depression are common psychiatric conditions after earthquakes. In these studies, the rates of PTSD and comorbid depression, respectively, were reported to be:
- 43% and 22% among survivors living in shelters 8 months post-disaster[3]

- 63% and 42% among treatment-seeking survivors 14 months post-disaster[4]
- 23% and 13% among survivors living in their homes in the epicentre region 14 months post-disaster[5]
- 39% and 18% among survivors living in shelters 20 months post-disaster.[6]

The most important risk factor for PTSD in these studies was greater intensity of fear during the earthquake.

These studies show that high exposure to earthquakes has long-term psychological effects, consistent with findings from other studies.[7–11]

Assessment of earthquake survivors

Effective post-earthquake mental health care programs require a screening instrument as a cost-effective means of identifying those in need of treatment. Few self-report measures of PTSD have been validated for use in developing countries and none of the existing measures are specific to earthquake trauma. A self-rated screening instrument for traumatic stress in earthquake survivors has, however, become available in recent years.[12] This scale, consisting of 17 PTSD and 6 depression items, estimates the diagnoses of PTSD and comorbid depression with a certainty of 81% and 77%, respectively.

Brief treatments for earthquake survivors

Given that large numbers of survivors may need help following major disasters, the treatment of choice needs to have the following characteristics:
- can be delivered within a short period of time
- proven to be effective
- easy to train professionals in its delivery
- feasible in post-disaster circumstances
- suitable for cost-effective dissemination to large numbers of survivors through media such as self-help manuals.

Among all treatments available for trauma survivors, cognitive–behavioral therapy (CBT) is the only one that comes close to meeting these criteria. Furthermore, our field surveys suggest that fear of earthquakes is the most important mediating factor in earthquake-related PTSD, and CBT is known to be highly effective in reducing conditioned fear and PTSD.[13] However, CBT is usually delivered in 8–10 sessions, and is therefore still not sufficiently brief in post-disaster circumstances. Shorter versions of CBT have recently been developed.

Modified behavioral treatment

Attempts have been made to shorten CBT without compromising its effectiveness by:

- limiting cognitive intervention to explanation of the treatment rationale only
- giving instructions for systematic exposure to feared and avoided situations
- shifting focus in treatment from a habituation rationale (e.g. 'stay in the situation until your anxiety subsides') to enhancement of sense of control over fear (e.g. 'stay in the situation until you feel in control over your fear').

The modified behavioral treatment was tested in a recent open clinical trial involving 231 survivors with chronic PTSD.[14] Strong treatment effects were observed in all measures of PTSD, depression and grief symptoms. After one treatment session, 76% of the survivors had improved; this increased to 88% after two sessions. Improvement was maintained at 3-month and 9-month follow-up.

Single-session behavioral treatment

Many earthquake survivors cannot attend treatment for more than one session because of disrupted life routines, demographic mobility and daily struggle for survival. A single-session modified behavioral treatment was therefore developed, which provided exposure instructions designed to enhance the individual's sense of control over feared situations. The effectiveness of this intervention has been tested in a randomized controlled trial involving 83 survivors with chronic PTSD.[15] The results show that the treatment is effective, leading to 75% improvement in PTSD symptoms in 3 months.

Highlights in **post-traumatic stress disorder after earthquakes** *2003–04*

WHAT'S IN?

- Brief assessment and treatment methods for earthquake survivors
- Cost-effective methods of treatment dissemination

WHAT'S NEW?

- A screening instrument for traumatic stress in earthquake survivors
- A two-session modified behavioral treatment program
- A single-session modified behavioral treatment
- A single-session behavioral treatment using an earthquake simulator
- A self-help manual for earthquake survivors

WHAT'S NEEDED?

- Controlled studies of modified behavioral treatment delivered through self-help manuals, video cassettes, computer programs, the Internet and television
- Controlled studies of the effectiveness of earthquake simulator-assisted exposure treatment in enhancing psychological preparedness for earthquakes
- Research on the effectiveness of modified behavioral treatment in other types of trauma

Behavioral treatment using an earthquake simulator

In an attempt to maximize the efficacy of single-session behavioral treatment, an additional behavioral intervention has been developed using an earthquake simulator. In a pilot study, 10 survivors with PTSD were given one session of exposure to simulated tremors, using an earthquake simulator that looked like a small house.[16] The patients could start and stop the tremors at any time and change their intensity by using a mobile control switch.

A substantial reduction in fear of earthquakes, and in PTSD and depression symptoms was noted at 6-week and 12-week follow-up. All patients reported reduction in distress associated with trauma-related memories. There was marked improvement in eight patients and slight improvement in the remaining two. The results suggest that the use of an earthquake simulator might significantly enhance the effectiveness of a behavioral program. The improved survivors reported that they no longer panicked during real earthquakes, suggesting that the treatment might also have a potential use in increasing psychological preparedness for earthquakes.

Dissemination of treatment

Dissemination of treatment to large numbers of survivors after natural disasters is a critical issue, particularly in developing countries with limited mental health care resources. Several cost-effective methods of dissemination are currently being considered. A highly structured self-help manual based on modified behavioral treatment principles was tested in a recent pilot study.[5] The study showed that when the manual is distributed to people with PTSD in the community, one in four people is likely to read it, follow the treatment instructions and improve.

Effective dissemination of treatment through computerized treatment programs, video cassettes, CDs, the Internet and television may also be possible, but further research is needed to examine the usefulness of such methods.

References

1. National Earthquake Information Center. Earthquakes with 1000 or more deaths from 1900. www.neic.cr.usgs.gov/neis/eqlists/eqsmajr.html (accessed 8 Dec 2003).

2. Norris FH, Friedman MJ, Watson PJ et al. 60,000 disaster victims speak: Part I. An empirical review of the empirical literature, 1981–2001. *Psychiatry* 2002; 65:207–39.

3. Başoğlu M, Şalcioğlu E, Livanou M. Traumatic stress responses in earthquake survivors in Turkey. *J Trauma Stress* 2002;15:269–76.

4. Livanou M, Başoğlu M, Şalcioğlu E, Kalender D. Traumatic stress responses in treatment-seeking earthquake survivors in Turkey. *J Nerv Ment Dis* 2002;190:816–23.

5. Başoğlu M, Kiliç C, Şalcioğlu E, Livanou M. Prevalence of post-traumatic stress disorder and comorbid depression in earthquake survivors in Turkey: an epidemiological study. *J Trauma Stress 2004;* in press.

6. Şalcioğlu E, Başoğlu M, Livanou M. Long-term psychological outcome in non-treatment-seeking earthquake survivors in Turkey. *J Nerv Ment Dis* 2003;191:154–60.

7. Armenian HK, Morikawa M, Melkonian AK et al. Loss as a determinant of PTSD in a cohort of adult survivors of the 1988 earthquake in Armenia: implications for policy. *Acta Psychiatr Scand* 2000;102:58–64.

8. Armenian HK, Morikawa M, Melkonian AK et al. Risk factors for depression in the survivors of the 1988 earthquake in Armenia. *J Urban Health* 2002;79:373–82.

9. Goenjian AK, Steinberg AM, Najarian LM et al. Prospective study of posttraumatic stress, anxiety, and depressive reactions after earthquake and political violence. *Am J Psychiatry* 2000;157:911–16.

10. McMillen JC, North CS, Smith EM. What parts of PTSD are normal: intrusion, avoidance, or arousal? Data from the Northridge, California, Earthquake. *J Trauma Stress* 2000;13:57–75.

11. Scott RL, Knoth RL, Beltran-Quiones M, Gomez N. Assessment of psychological functioning in adolescent earthquake victims in Colombia using the MMPI-A. *J Trauma Stress* 2003;16:49–57.

12. Başoğlu M, Şalcioğlu E, Livanou M et al. A study of the validity of a screening instrument for traumatic stress in earthquake survivors in Turkey. *J Trauma Stress* 2001; 14:491–509.

13. Livanou M. Psychological treatments for post-traumatic stress disorder: an overview. *Int Rev Psychiatry* 2001;13:181–8.

14. Başoğlu M, Livanou M, Şalcioğlu E, Kalender D. A brief behavioural treatment of chronic posttraumatic stress disorder in earthquake survivors: results from an open clinical trial. *Psychol Med* 2003; 33:647–54.

15. Başoğlu M, Şalcioğlu E, Livanou M et al. The effectiveness of a single session behavioral treatment in PTSD: preliminary findings from a controlled clinical trial. Presented at the Spring Symposia, Antalya, Turkey, 24–26 April 2002.

16. Başoğlu M, Livanou M, Şalcioğlu E. A single session exposure treatment of traumatic stress in earthquake survivors using an earthquake simulator. *Am J Psychiatry* 2003;160:788–90.

Unexplained fatigue symptoms and syndromes

Petros Skapinakis MD MPH PhD **and Glyn Lewis** FRCPsych PhD
Department of Psychiatry, University of Bristol, UK

Fatigue is a common symptom in the community, with up to 25% of the general population reporting substantial fatigue of at least 2 weeks' duration.[1] It is also a common complaint in primary care, with 10–30% of patients reporting fatigue, although it is less commonly a presenting complaint.[2] Fatigue of less than 1 month's duration (acute fatigue, Table 1) is more likely to be a secondary symptom of an established medical condition. Chronic fatigue (lasting longer than 6 months) is more likely to be a medically unexplained symptom.

Chronic unexplained fatigue is considered to be the main symptom of various syndromes, including chronic fatigue syndrome (CFS) and neurasthenia (a condition included in ICD-10 as a neurotic disorder).

This chapter reviews key papers in the field of chronic fatigue that were published in 2002 or 2003 and cited in MEDLINE or the Cochrane library. The search terms used to identify these papers were chronic fatigue syndrome, chronic fatigue, idiopathic fatigue, unexplained fatigue, prolonged fatigue, and neurasthenia.

Epidemiology of chronic fatigue and chronic fatigue syndrome

Unexplained chronic fatigue in adults is relatively common, with a prevalence in the community of 2–9%.[1] In contrast, the prevalence of CFS is much lower, ranging from 0.007% to 0.6%.[2]

Epidemiological data for chronic fatigue in children and adolescents are relatively sparse, but the results of a well-conducted UK study have recently been published.[3] The researchers interviewed a representative sample of 4240 children and adolescents aged

TABLE 1

Definitions

Acute fatigue
Fatigue of < 1 month's duration

Prolonged fatigue
Fatigue of ≥ 1 month's duration

Chronic unexplained fatigue
A subset of prolonged fatigue, defined as fatigue of ≥ 6 months' duration, with other known medical conditions excluded by clinical diagnosis.

Chronic fatigue syndrome
According to the Centers for Disease Control and Prevention definition (1994), both of the following criteria must generally be met in order to make a diagnosis of chronic fatigue syndrome

- The patient must have severe chronic unexplained fatigue (≥ 6 months' duration),
- Concurrently, the patient must have four or more of the following symptoms:
    - substantial impairment in short-term memory or concentration
    - sore throat
    - tender lymph nodes
    - muscle pain
    - multi-joint pain without swelling or redness
    - headaches of a new type, pattern or severity
    - unrefreshing sleep
    - post-exertional malaise lasting more than 24 hours

The symptoms must have persisted or recurred for 6 or more consecutive months of illness and must not have predated the fatigue

(CONTINUED)

TABLE 1 (CONTINUED)

Neurasthenia

According to ICD-10, neurasthenia is an unexplained fatigue syndrome of at least 3 months' duration, which additionally requires the following criteria

- At least one of the following symptoms must be present:
  - feelings of muscular aches and pains
  - dizziness
  - tension headaches
  - sleep disturbance
  - inability to relax
  - irritability
- The disorder does not occur in the presence of mood disorders, panic disorder, generalized anxiety disorder, post-concussional syndrome, post-encephalitic syndrome or organic emotionally labile syndrome

11–15 years and living in private households in the UK. They found the prevalence for chronic fatigue was 0.57% (95% confidence interval: 0.34–0.80) and that for CFS was 0.19% (95% confidence interval: 0.06–0.32). Therefore, it seems that chronic fatigue, and possibly CFS, is less common in children or adolescents compared with adults. An interesting finding of this study was that parental report of myalgic encephalomyelitis or CFS was very rare. Only 4 of 10 438 mothers reported that their child suffered from either of these syndromes.

Most of the epidemiological studies of fatigue have been conducted in developed Western countries. A recent study has provided data on the prevalence of unexplained fatigue and related syndromes in several countries with different levels of economic development.[4] This study found that the prevalence of self-reported chronic fatigue was higher in subjects living in developed countries such as the UK, Germany, the Netherlands and France, compared with those living in less developed countries such as Nigeria, China and India. In contrast, fatigue was more common as a presenting complaint in primary care patients living in less developed countries.

An interesting finding from the same study was that the association between fatigue and psychiatric morbidity appears to be stronger in developing countries than in developed countries. The authors conclude that in developing countries fatigue may be an indicator of hidden psychiatric morbidity, while in more highly developed countries fatigue may be a symbol of psychosocial distress, which does not often lead to consultation behavior.

Diagnostic factors

Most definitions of chronic fatigue and related syndromes have been developed by expert consensus. However, these definitions have been criticized. One major criticism is that a clear distinction is implied between severe CFS (defined on the basis of additional physical or cognitive symptoms; see Table 1) and the less severe form of 'idiopathic' or chronic fatigue.[5]

In 2003, several studies were published that attempted to evaluate the validity of this distinction by comparing subjects with CFS and subjects with chronic fatigue only. Evengard et al. studied CFS patients in an infectious diseases clinic in Sweden, and observed that these individuals were more likely to report other somatic symptoms, to have an acute infectious onset and to be less psychologically disturbed compared with subjects with chronic fatigue only.[6] However, this was a highly selected sample and selection bias is very likely.

Studies in primary care are more useful in this respect. A study in the UK investigated 141 patients who presented to their primary care physician with chronic unexplained fatigue as the main symptom. Almost 70% of patients had chronic fatigue and not CFS. Patients meeting the criteria for CFS were more disabled, consulted their primary care physician more often, had more associated symptoms and were twice as likely to be depressed.[7]

In another study in primary care, the authors analyzed data from 14 countries and reported that subjects with more severe forms of fatigue were more likely to suffer from psychiatric disorders. The prevalence of depression in subjects meeting criteria for unexplained fatigue but not CFS was 47%, compared with a figure of 61% in those meeting CFS criteria.[8]

Therefore, it appears that the criterion relating to symptoms in the 1994 Centers for Disease Control and Prevention definition of CFS artificially selects subjects with more psychological distress, mainly because of the well-established association between multiple somatic symptoms and psychiatric disorders. Future revisions of the CFS definition should take this into account, perhaps either by removing this criterion or by selecting a subset of the current symptoms that is both useful and more specific for CFS.

Relation to psychiatric morbidity

The most controversial area in the field of unexplained fatigue syndromes is the strong association with common psychiatric conditions, especially depression and anxiety disorders. In the community, about 40% of subjects with chronic fatigue may also have a common psychiatric condition.[1] This comorbidity is increased in primary care, where more than 50% of patients with unexplained fatigue may also meet the criteria for depression and anxiety.[8] As mentioned above, this association is even stronger in CFS patients, with more than 80% in an international primary care study also suffering from either depression or generalized anxiety disorder.[8]

Possible explanations for this association include the following:
- psychiatric disorders are secondary to CFS, which is a disabling condition of unknown etiology
- psychiatric disorders are causing fatigue syndromes in predisposed individuals
- unknown confounding factors cause this association
- it is the artificial result of overlapping operational definitions.

It is worth noting that these explanations are not mutually exclusive and may all explain a small part of the reported strong association.

A twin study published in 2002 did not find evidence for genetic covariation between fatigue and psychiatric conditions in 69 monozygotic and 31 dizygotic female twin pairs, with only one co-twin reporting chronic fatigue.[9] The authors concluded that these findings support the view that the association is due to environmental factors or overlapping definitions.

The issue of causality or reverse causality (the first and second of the points listed above) requires longitudinal studies and these are sparse, especially studies involving unselected community or primary care samples. In a secondary analysis, Skapinakis et al. have examined the temporal relationship between unexplained fatigue syndromes and psychiatric disorders in an international study in primary care.[10] At 12-month follow-up in subjects free of psychiatric disease at baseline, fatigue was found to increase the risk of developing a new episode of a psychiatric disorder, while psychiatric disorders increased the risk of a new episode of fatigue among subjects who were free of fatigue at baseline. Therefore, the strong cross-sectional association is more likely to be the result of confounding factors or overlapping definitions. However, the possibility exists that both conditions are independent risk factors for each other. A possible mediating mechanism may be the level of physical activity, a factor that should be investigated in future studies.[11]

Other etiologic factors

Little progress has been made regarding the role of other biological or psychosocial factors in the etiology of chronic fatigue and CFS. Although the role of genetic factors is not clear, findings of a recent study of a community sample of twins suggest that genetic factors are more important in women and environmental factors are more important in men.[12]

There is some evidence for a reduced cortisol output in some patients, but a recent review on the neuroendocrinology of chronic fatigue concluded that there is no evidence of a specific or uniform dysfunction of the hypothalamic–pituitary–adrenal axis in CFS patients.[13]

A recent study has found that CFS patients are more likely to attribute their functional somatic symptoms to a physical illness than are non-fatigued controls.[14]

Highlights in **unexplained fatigue symptoms and syndromes** 2003–04

WHAT'S IN?

- Chronic fatigue syndrome (CFS) is uncommon in children and is associated with a better prognosis, compared with adults
- Unexplained fatigue syndromes are more common in countries with a higher level of economic development, but fatigue as a presenting complaint is more common in countries with a lower level of development
- Genetic factors may be more important in the etiology of chronic fatigue in women, while environmental factors may be more important in men
- The prognosis for adults with unexplained fatigue syndromes may be better than previously thought

WHAT'S OUT?

- The poor prognosis for CFS patients

WHAT'S CONTROVERSIAL?

- The relationship between CFS and psychiatric disorders
- Pharmacological intervention

Prognosis and prognostic factors

Several studies on the prognosis or natural history of unexplained fatigue syndromes have been published in the past 2 years. A retrospective survey, involving 36 children with a diagnosis of CFS who were attending a primary care specialist interest clinic, confirmed the relatively good prognosis of CFS in children. Most of the children (29 of 36) returned to normal health or improved significantly over time.[15]

The prognosis of adult patients attending tertiary centers is generally poor. However, a study in the Netherlands reported that CFS patients with a short duration of illness (less than 2 years) had a better prognosis than those with a longer duration of illness (46% improved at 12 months versus 20%).[16]

In the primary care setting, an international study in 14 countries reported a very good prognosis for unexplained fatigue syndromes in adults, with fewer than 20% of subjects having a persistent unexplained fatigue syndrome over 12-months' follow-up, with small differences among the countries.[17]

The most significant predictor of a poor prognosis in patients with CFS or chronic fatigue is the severity of fatigue,[18] followed by the presence of comorbid psychiatric disorders[17] and a physical illness attribution.[19]

Treatment

Data on the efficacy of pharmacological intervention for CFS and related syndromes continue to be inconclusive. In a crossover trial, citalopram, a selective serotonin-reuptake inhibitor, was found to reduce fatigue significantly in 31 patients with chronic unexplained fatigue; however, the small sample size and the short duration of placebo use (1 week) limit the interpretation of these results.[20] Similarly, a small randomized controlled trial of the effectiveness of dexamphetamine in patients with CFS found a significant effect in favor of the active treatment, but the small number of patients (10 in each group) is a serious limitation.[21]

Regarding non-pharmacological treatment, a systematic review of interventions available for patients with common somatic syndromes confirmed that cognitive–behavioral therapy is an effective and acceptable treatment for chronic fatigue.[22]

References

1. Skapinakis P, Lewis G, Meltzer H. Clarifying the relationship between unexplained chronic fatigue and psychiatric morbidity: results from a community survey in Great Britain. *Am J Psychiatry* 2000;157:1492–8.

2. Afari N, Buchwald D. Chronic fatigue syndrome: a review. *Am J Psychiatry* 2003;160:221–36.

3. Chalder T, Goodman R, Wessely S et al. Epidemiology of chronic fatigue syndrome and self-reported myalgic encephalomyelitis in 5–15-year-olds: cross-sectional study. *BMJ* 2003;327:654–5.

4. Skapinakis P, Lewis G, Mavreas V. Cross-cultural differences in the epidemiology of unexplained fatigue syndromes in primary care. *Br J Psychiatry* 2003;182:205–9.

5. Fukuda K, Straus SE, Hickie I et al. The chronic fatigue syndrome: a comprehensive approach to its definition and study. International Chronic Fatigue Syndrome Study Group. *Ann Intern Med* 1994;121:953–9.

6. Evengard B, Jonzon E, Sandberg A et al. Differences between patients with chronic fatigue syndrome and with chronic fatigue at an infectious disease clinic in Stockholm, Sweden. *Psychiatry Clin Neurosci* 2003;57:361–8.

7. Darbishire L, Ridsdale L, Seed PT. Distinguishing patients with chronic fatigue from those with chronic fatigue syndrome: a diagnostic study in UK primary care. *Br J Gen Pract* 2003;53:441–5.

8. Skapinakis P, Lewis G, Mavreas V. Unexplained fatigue syndromes in a multinational primary care sample: specificity of definition and prevalence and distinctiveness from depression and generalized anxiety. *Am J Psychiatry* 2003;160:785–7.

9. Roy-Byrne P, Afari N, Ashton S et al. Chronic fatigue and anxiety/depression: a twin study. *Br J Psychiatry* 2002;180:29–34.

10. Skapinakis P, Lewis G, Mavreas V. Temporal relations between unexplained fatigue and depression: longitudinal data from an international study in primary care. *Psychosom Med* 2004;(in press).

11. White PD. The role of physical inactivity in the chronic fatigue syndrome. *J Psychosom Res* 2000;49:283–4.

12. Sullivan PF, Kovalenko P, York TP et al. Fatigue in a community sample of twins. *Psychol Med* 2003;33:263–81.

13. Cleare AJ. The neuroendocrinology of chronic fatigue syndrome. *Endocr Rev* 2003;24:236–52.

14. Butler JA, Chalder T, Wessely S. Causal attributions for somatic sensations in patients with chronic fatigue syndrome and their partners. *Psychol Med* 2001;31:97–105.

15. Patel MX, Smith DG, Chalder T et al. Chronic fatigue syndrome in children: a cross-sectional survey. *Arch Dis Child* 2003;88:894–8.

16. van der Werf SP, de Vree B, Alberts M et al. Natural course and predicting self-reported improvement in patients with chronic fatigue syndrome with a relatively short illness duration. *J Psychosom Res* 2002;53:749–53.

17. Skapinakis P, Lewis G, Mavreas V. One-year outcome of unexplained fatigue syndromes in primary care: results from an international study. *Psychol Med* 2003;33:857–66.

18. Taylor RR, Jason LA, Curie CJ. Prognosis of chronic fatigue in a community-based sample. *Psychosom Med* 2002;64:319–27.

19. Chalder T, Godfrey E, Ridsdale L et al. Predictors of outcome in a fatigued population in primary care following a randomized controlled trial. *Psychol Med* 2003;33:283–7.

20. Hartz AJ, Bentler SE, Brake KA et al. The effectiveness of citalopram for idiopathic chronic fatigue. *J Clin Psychiatry* 2003;64:927–35.

21. Olson LG, Ambrogetti A, Sutherland DC. A pilot randomized controlled trial of dexamphetamine in patients with chronic fatigue syndrome. *Psychosomatics* 2003;44:38–43.

22. Raine R, Haines A, Sensky T et al. Systematic review of mental health interventions for patients with common somatic symptoms: can research evidence from secondary care be extrapolated to primary care? *BMJ* 2002;325:1082–93.

Cancer and mood disorders

Laura K Sherman MD and Michael J Fisch MD MPH
Department of Neuro-oncology, and Department of Palliative Care and Rehabilitation Medicine, University of Texas MD Anderson Cancer Center, Houston, USA

Epidemiology and etiology

Depression is the most prevalent mood disorder among patients with cancer, with a median point prevalence in a recent literature review of 22–29%.[1] The prevalence may vary by tumor site, with the highest prevalence (50%) in pancreatic cancer.[2] Full-blown depressive illness is not a 'normal' response to cancer, and it is critical that the depression is diagnosed and treated, because it can impact on both quality of life and mortality.[3] One recent large study of more than 20 000 Danish breast cancer patients has shown depression to be a negative prognostic factor for breast cancer mortality.[4]

Previous research has found that the most common mood disorder in the cancer population is adjustment disorder,[5] commonly referred to as a reactive depression, suggesting that pathogenesis of the symptoms relates to patients' aberrant adjustment to the stressor. A recent groundbreaking study has demonstrated that inherited genetic differences in serotonin transporter promoter alleles are associated with an individual's risk of developing depression in response to environmental stressors.[6]

Other new etiologies for depressive illness specifically in the cancer population have also been explored recently. New developments in psychoneuroimmunology suggest that activation of inflammatory cytokines may lead to behavioral changes, thus inducing depressive illnesses and 'sickness behavior' in this population.[7] Higher than normal plasma interleukin-6 concentrations have been shown to be associated with major depression in cancer patients, and this finding is being actively investigated. Furthermore, hormonal etiologies for depression in particular cancers have been suggested, such as depression induced by chemical menopause in patients with breast cancer,[8] or by androgen ablation in patients with prostate cancer.[9]

Diagnosis

Diagnosing depressive illness in patients with cancer can be difficult, as the cancer itself or side effects of treatment may account for many symptoms relating to the autonomic nervous system, such as changes in weight or energy level. Identifying the more cognitive symptoms of depression, such as anhedonia, indecisiveness, suicidal ideation, guilt, and feelings of hopelessness and helplessness, is very important. Furthermore, a distinction must be made from the normal grieving process.

A syndrome that incorporates classic cognitive symptoms with autonomic nervous system symptoms of depression, which is persistent for 2 weeks or more and which causes impairment of functioning, is most likely depression. The National Cancer Institute (NCI) has developed a comprehensive list of risk factors, which may help to alert the clinician to patients at risk for depressive illness (Table 1).

Other factors that can complicate a diagnosis of depression are comorbid medical conditions that mimic or induce depression, as well as depression-inducing drugs commonly used in the cancer population. These potential etiologies or confounders should always be considered when assessing a patient for depressive illness (Tables 2 and 3).

Screening for major depression can be time-consuming. Screening tools may therefore be helpful; both the Psychological Distress Inventory[10] and the Hospital Anxiety and Depression Scale[11] have been validated in the cancer population.

Treatment

Although depression is difficult to diagnose in the cancer population, it is highly treatable[12] and aggressive treatment positively impacts on quality of life, morbidity and mortality. The

TABLE 1

Risk factors for depression in patients with cancer

Cancer-related risk factors
- Depression at the time of cancer diagnosis
- Poorly controlled pain
- Advanced stage of cancer
- Additional concurrent life stressors
- Increased physical impairment or discomfort
- Pancreatic cancer
- Being unmarried together with having head/neck cancer
- Treatment with certain chemotherapeutic agents

Non-cancer-related risk factors
- History of depression
  - Two or more episodes in a lifetime
  - First episode early or late in life
- Lack of family support
- Family history of depression or suicide
- Previous suicide attempt(s)
- History of alcoholism or drug abuse
- Concurrent illnesses that produce depressive symptoms
- Past treatment for psychological problems

Source: National Cancer Institute, 2003[20]

combined modalities of support, psychotherapy and antidepressants should be offered to patients whose depressive symptoms impair their functioning.

Non-pharmacological interventions. Most research on the treatment of mood disorders and mood symptoms in the cancer population has focused on non-pharmacological interventions, which have typically been tested in mildly emotionally distressed individuals

TABLE 2
Medical illnesses that can mimic or induce depression

- Grief
- Uncontrolled pain
- Delirium
- Dementia
- Electrolyte/metabolic abnormalities
- Stroke
- Brain metastasis
- Hypothyroidism (especially radiation-induced)

TABLE 3
Commonly used oncology drugs associated with depression

- Interferon-α
- Interleukin-2
- Corticosteroids
- Procarbazine
- Tamoxifen
- L-asparaginase
- Leuprolide
- Amphotericin B
- Vincristine
- Vinblastine

versus patients with full-blown depressive disorders. The preponderance of evidence points to the importance of good social support and beneficial effects of both individual and group psychotherapy. A recent study demonstrated a strong inverse relationship between social support and psychiatric morbidity in patients with early-stage breast cancer.[13]

Highlights in cancer and mood disorders 2003–04

WHAT'S IN?

- Consideration of biological etiologies of depression in cancer
- Treatment with both antidepressants and psychotherapy/support
- Tailoring antidepressants to address somatic symptoms
- Use of selective serotonin reuptake inhibitors, mirtazapine, venlafaxine and bupropion

WHAT'S OUT?

- Assuming that a new depression in a cancer patient is an adjustment disorder
- Treatment with only psychotherapy/support
- Tricyclic antidepressants and monoamine oxidase inhibitors

WHAT'S EMERGING?

- Prevention of depression and other physical symptoms with antidepressants
- Multidisciplinary treatment of depression in the cancer population

Antidepressant agents. Although there is a paucity of controlled trials of antidepressants for depression in the cancer population, the available evidence suggests this class of drugs is effective in the medically ill, including those with cancer.[14]

The NCI advocates that when adjustment symptoms significantly interfere with a person's functioning, the patient should be treated for major depression.[13] Certainly, when a patient with cancer meets the full criteria for major depression, treatment with psychotherapeutic modalities and antidepressants should be considered.

In the cancer population, selective serotonin reuptake inhibitors (SSRIs), such as citalopram, escitalopram, fluoxetine, fluvoxamine, paroxetine and sertraline, and the newer generation non-SSRI drugs, such as mirtazapine, venlafaxine, nefazodone and bupropion, are commonly used to treat depression. Tricyclic antidepressants and monoamine oxidase inhibitors (MAOIs) are less commonly used in this group of patients because of their side-effect profiles and potential drug interactions.

Care should always be used when selecting an antidepressant in order to avoid P450 liver enzyme interactions and other drug interactions (e.g. concomitant administration with a non-antidepressant MAOI, such as the chemotherapeutic agent procarbazine or the antibacterial linezolid; this combination can precipitate serotonin syndrome as well as hypertensive crisis). If the patient has hepatic or renal impairment, it is important to initiate antidepressant drugs at a low dose and titrate the dose slowly. Bupropion, which is also indicated for nicotine dependence, should be avoided in patients with a history of seizures.

A recent trend in antidepressant prescribing in the cancer population has been to address physical symptoms in addition to depressive symptoms. It has been suggested that citalopram is effective for both depression and hot flashes in patients with breast cancer who have undergone chemical menopause.[9] Two previous studies have shown that the serotonergic antidepressants paroxetine[15] and venlafaxine[16] are efficacious for hot flashes. Mirtazapine has efficacy for multiple somatic symptoms, including pain, nausea and poor appetite.[17]

A similar recent trend in antidepressant prescribing in patients with cancer has been to address psychological variables other than depression alone. Several studies have looked at the impact of antidepressants on the quality of life in patients with cancer. The most recent study, a double-blind trial comparing fluoxetine with placebo, demonstrated an improved quality of life and reduced depressive symptoms in the group receiving fluoxetine.[18]

Drug-induced depression can be treated with antidepressants

without necessarily having to reduce the dose of, or discontinue, a potentially life-saving chemotherapeutic drug. A recent groundbreaking study has demonstrated that depression induced by high-dose interferon-α can be prevented by paroxetine.[19]

References

1. Hotopf M, Addington-Hall J, Ly KL. Depression in advanced disease: a systemic review. Part 1: prevalence and case finding. *Palliat Med* 2002;16:81–97.

2. Newport DJ, Nemeroff CB. Treatment of depression in the cancer patient. *Clin Geriat* 1999;7:40–55.

3. Loberiza FR, Rizzo JD, Bredeson CN et al. Association of depressive syndrome and early deaths among patients after stem-cell transplantation for malignant diseases. *J Clin Oncol* 2002;8:2118–26.

4. Hjerl K, Andersen E, Keiding N et al. Depression as a prognostic factor for breast cancer mortality. *Psychosomatics* 2003;44:24–30.

5. Derogatis LR, Morrow GR, Fetting J et al. The prevalence of psychiatric disorders among cancer patients. *JAMA* 1983;249:751–7.

6. Caspi A, Sugden K, Moffit T et al. Influence of life stress on depression: moderation by a polymorphism in the 5-HTT gene. *Science* 2003;301:386–9.

7. Raison CL, Miller AH. Depression and cancer: new developments regarding diagnosis and treatment. *Biol Psychiatry* 2003;54:283–94.

8. Musselman DL, Miller AH, Porter MR et al. Higher than normal plasma interleukin-6 concentrations in cancer patients with depression: preliminary findings. *Am J Psychiatry* 2001;158:1252–7.

9. Sherman LK. Citalopram treatment of chemical menopause induced depression and hot flashes in breast cancer patients (abstract). *Psychooncology* 2003;12(suppl):S158. Presented at the 2003 World Congress of Psychooncology, Banff, Alberta, Canada, 25 April 2003.

10. Pirl WF, Siegel GI, Goode MJ et al. Depression in men receiving androgen deprivation therapy for prostate cancer: a pilot study. *Psychooncology* 2002;6;518–23.

11. Morasso G, Costantini M, Baracco G et al. Assessing psychological distress in cancer patients: validation of a self-administered questionnaire. *Oncology* 1996;53:295–302.

12. Zigmond AS, Snaith RP. The hospital anxiety and depression scale. *Acta Psychiatr Scand* 1983;67:361–70.

13. National Cancer Institute. Depression (PDQ): the health professional version. 2003. www.cancer.gov/cancerinfo/pdq/supportivecare/depression/HealthProfessional

14. Simpson SJ, Carlson LE, Beck CA et al. Effects of a brief intervention on social support and psychiatric morbidity in breast cancer patients. *Psychooncology* 2002;11:282–94.

15. Haig RA. Management of depression in patients with advanced cancer. *Med J Aus* 1992;156: 499–503.

16. Stearns V, Issacs C, Rowland J et al. A pilot trial assessing the efficacy of paroxetine hydrochloride in controlling hot flashes in breast cancer survivors. *Ann Oncol* 2000;11:17–22.

17. Loprinzi CL, Kugler JW, Sloan JA et al. Venlafaxine in management of hot flashes in survivors of breast cancer: a randomized controlled trial. *Lancet* 2000;356:2059–63.

18. Theobald DE, Kirsh KL, Holtsclaw E et al. An open-label, crossover trial of mirtazapine (15 and 30 mg) in cancer patients with pain and other distressing symptoms. *J Pain Symptom Manage* 2002; 23:442–7.

19. Fisch MJ, Loehrer PJ, Kristeller J et al. Fluoxetine versus placebo in advanced cancer outpatients: a double-blinded trial of the Hoosier Oncology Group. *J Clin Oncol* 2003;21:1937–43.

20. Theobald DE, Kirsh KL, Holtsclaw E et al. An open label pilot study of citalopram for depression and boredom in ambulatory cancer patients. *Palliat Supp Care* 2003; 1:71–7.

21. Musselman DL, Lawson DH, Gumnick JF et al. Paroxetine for the prevention of depression induced by high-dose interferon alfa. *N Engl J Med* 2001;344:961–6.

Asperger's syndrome

Jan Blacher PhD and Rachel M Fenning
University of California, Graduate School of Education, Riverside and University of California, Los Angeles, USA

Asperger's syndrome was first described by Hans Asperger in 1944, and has since become the subject of numerous research and clinical studies. Individuals with Asperger's syndrome have impaired social abilities, but unimpaired or occasionally superior language skills and intellectual functioning.[1,2]

Once considered rare, the prevalence of Asperger's syndrome has recently been reported to be as high as 1 in 500, with 1 in 350 children considered to have either pervasive developmental disorder or Asperger's syndrome.[3] Frombonne, however, puts the rate much lower, at 2.5/10,000.[4] Even at this rate, meeting current and future treatment needs is problematic.

Differential diagnosis

Although Asperger's syndrome is recognized as a separate disorder in the DSM-IV and ICD-10, the validity of the diagnostic distinction between Asperger's syndrome and high functioning autism (HFA) remains controversial. Many consider the DSM-IV and ICD-10 criteria for Asperger's syndrome to be too narrow, making a formal diagnosis of Asperger's syndrome unlikely, given the requirement that a diagnosis of autism take precedence.[3,5–7] As a consequence, researchers often devise independent definitions of Asperger's syndrome, which reduces comparability across studies, complicates analyses of outcome and yields inconclusive results.[6]

Recent investigations emphasize outcome in order to justify differential diagnosis between Asperger's syndrome and HFA. Several studies have affirmed differences in adaptive and behavioral outcomes in childhood. Individuals with Asperger's syndrome demonstrate higher functioning across core domains and less severe or fewer symptoms than those with HFA.[8,9] In addition, the presence of early language skills, although an important factor affecting outcome in children with Asperger's syndrome, functions as a particularly significant predictor of later functioning in children with HFA.[7] Such findings have led some investigators to postulate the existence of different determinants of outcome for these two disorders, but additional research is necessary.[7]

An alternative perspective suggests that initial differences in symptom presentation between Asperger's syndrome and HFA may ultimately converge as individuals with HFA develop greater language skills over time.[7-9] Evidence that children with Asperger's syndrome continue to experience difficulties in social interaction, despite early or age-appropriate language acquisition and use, supports this hypothesis. Howlin also found that individuals with Asperger's syndrome often do not maintain early levels of language proficiency and instead demonstrate below average language abilities in adulthood. The results of this study also indicate that other initial group differences between people with HFA and Asperger's syndrome may decrease over time, particularly in the domains of social functioning and communication. Given the relative lack of substantial differences in adult functioning within her sample, Howlin questions the clinical utility of distinguishing between Asperger's syndrome and HFA.[5]

Other research has focused more specifically on core characteristics that differentiate Asperger's syndrome from HFA, rather than focusing on outcome. For instance, Klin and Volkmar review evidence indicating that individuals diagnosed with Asperger's syndrome demonstrate a profile consistent with a non-verbal learning disability, whereas those with HFA show a profile defined by strengths in non-verbal skills.[6] Findings also suggest that children with Asperger's syndrome may produce more speech assertions characterized by explanations and internal state language than children diagnosed with HFA.[10]

Past research and current diagnostic criteria have identified motor clumsiness as a feature associated with Asperger's syndrome, but not HFA.[6] However, recent comparative research has not found differences in this characteristic.[5]

The diagnostic distinction between Asperger's syndrome and HFA therefore remains tentative, and further research is required before definitive conclusions can be drawn. Improvements in diagnostic consistency, appropriate group matching and larger sample sizes, as well as enhanced understanding of etiologic differences, will facilitate much needed clarification in this area.[5-9]

Core characteristics

Social impairments are hallmark characteristics of Asperger's syndrome.[6] However, unlike individuals with HFA, people with Asperger's syndrome typically desire social contact but demonstrate a degree of social ineptitude that often results in isolation.[6,9] Rule-oriented and formulistic in social interactions,[6,11] individuals with Asperger's syndrome struggle with abstract concepts such as humor[12] and have trouble understanding others' perspectives.[13] They often fail to form close relationships.[5] Indeed, as the importance of interpersonal relationships increases during later childhood and adolescence, many individuals with Asperger's syndrome have trouble adapting to heightened expectations and may experience greater social difficulties over time.[3,8]

Common features of Asperger's syndrome include poor prosody[6,14] and neglecting to adjust the rate of speech or volume appropriately.[6] Difficulties in understanding, discriminating between or employing appropriate intonation may stem from deficits in auditory sensory processing, particularly in sound-feature encoding and sound discrimination.[14] However, Asperger's syndrome is also associated with weak conversational skills characterized by inattention to listeners' needs. Individuals with Asperger's syndrome often dominate discussions by focusing on restricted patterns of interest[8] and may overemphasize references to internal states of desire relative to personal thoughts or beliefs about others.[10] Those with Asperger's syndrome also demonstrate circumscribed deficits in episodic memory, including increased reliance on familiar experiences rather than recollection.[16]

Storytelling abilities may be deficient in people with Asperger's syndrome, with these individuals identifying fewer causal explanations in personal and storybook narratives, and using less complex syntax in personal accounts than individuals with HFA.[15]

Deficits in face perception may further contribute to the social interaction difficulties of those with Asperger's syndrome. Although most studies do not differentiate between HFA and Asperger's syndrome, findings suggest that those with autism spectrum disorder demonstrate pervasive face-perception abnormalities, including selective deficits in face recognition that do not extend to non-face objects.[17] Individuals with autism spectrum disorder demonstrate diminished activation in the fusiform gyrus while viewing faces, and increased activation in brain areas typically associated with object recognition.[17,18] They are also less susceptible to the face inversion effect (they have markedly less difficulty in recognizing upside-down faces than do subjects with normal or typical development),[17,19] and tend to focus on the lower parts of the face, particularly the mouth, to extrapolate social meaning.[17,20]

Comorbidity

Although studies tend to combine analyses of individuals with HFA and Asperger's syndrome, findings suggest strong comorbidity between Asperger's syndrome and psychiatric disorders, including mood, anxiety, attention, aggression and obsessional problems.[3,6,11] Neurotransmitter system deficits may partly account for the prominence of anxiety and depressive symptoms.[11] However, heightened vulnerability to anxiety may also relate to self-awareness among those with Asperger's syndrome, and an associated sensitivity to social frustrations, failures and rejection.[3]

Heredity and family patterns

Few family aggregation studies have focused specifically on Asperger's syndrome, but relevant research suggests the presence of social disabilities among relatives, especially males, of individuals diagnosed with Asperger's syndrome.[6] There is also evidence to suggest that people with autism or Asperger's syndrome and their

Highlights in Asperger's syndrome 2003–2004

WHAT'S IN?

- Interventions that focus on specific aspects of social communication
- Recognition of Asperger's syndrome as a possibly distinct disorder (as defined in DSM-IV and ICD-10), thus promoting further research
- Prevalence estimates of Asperger's syndrome of at least 1 in 500; 1 in 350 have either Asperger's syndrome or PDD-NOS (pervasive developmental disorder – not otherwise specified)
- Examination of outcomes to determine differential diagnosis of high functioning autism and Asperger's syndrome

WHAT'S NEW?

- Use of oxytocin for the reduction of repetitive behaviors in Asperger's syndrome
- Concept of different developmental trajectories for autism spectrum disorder and Asperger's syndrome
- More innovative behavioral strategies for stress management and social interventions

immediate family members may display abnormalities in plasma amino acid levels, suggesting an inherited vulnerability to biochemical dysfunction.[21] Family environment, though not the cause of Asperger's syndrome, may affect the course of the disorder. As has been found in children with intellectual disability,[22] family processes may influence the development of comorbid behavior problems. Conversely, a child with Asperger's syndrome may negatively impact family dynamics by contributing to increased familial stress.[9]

Treatment

The main treatments for Asperger's syndrome are behavioral and pharmacological. Typically, interventions target aspects of social

WHAT'S PROBLEMATIC?

- Differential diagnosis (Asperger's syndrome as distinct from HFA)
- Studies with small sample sizes and heterogeneous populations
- Costs and/or availability limits accessibility of interventions (behavioral or pharmacological) for individuals with Asperger's syndrome and their families

WHAT'S MISSING?

- Studies of Asperger's syndrome across individuals' lifetimes, especially at adolescence
- Focus on outcomes specifically in Asperger's syndrome (as opposed to autism in general)
- Research on the impact of Asperger's syndrome on families (mothers, fathers, siblings)
- Research on family processes that affect the course of Asperger's syndrome

understanding, social cognition or emotions.[22] One recent review covers stress management for individuals with Asperger's syndrome,[23] and includes descriptions of strategies to increase social understanding, such as 'cartooning' (using comic strip conversations to analyze social scripts), 'social autopsies' (analyzing recent social situations in order to understand social mistakes), sensory awareness and self-awareness. Direct instruction in the specific social area of concern appears to be most effective.[23,24] Behavioral treatments also work well if they involve peers, and if the child with Asperger's syndrome has the opportunity to practice newly learned skills in varied, naturalistic environments.

Ultimately, the establishment of more detailed diagnostic criteria and better evaluation methods is likely to improve the treatment of Asperger's syndrome.[24] The identification of molecular and neurobiological mechanisms underlying Asperger's syndrome, either through detailed gene expression profiling or the analysis of expressed proteins, will also help to pinpoint the best treatment, especially if medications are involved.[25] Some core symptoms of autism have been reduced through psychopharmacological treatment. Recently, oxytocin infusions were shown to decrease negative, repetitive behaviors in adults with a diagnosis of either autism or Asperger's syndrome, compared with placebo.[26] In addition, research on patterns of family life could contribute to an understanding of Asperger's syndrome, with potentially significant influence on diagnosis and treatment.

Acknowledgements

The preparation of this manuscript was supported in part by NICHD Grant Number RO1HD21324 (J Blacher, PI) and NICHD Grant Number 34879-1459 (K Crnic, PI; BL Baker, J Blacher, C Edelbrock, co-PIs). The authors would like to thank Monica Schalow of the University of California, Riverside Families Project for her research assistance.

References

1. Wing L. Asperger's syndrome: a clinical account. *Psychol Med* 1981;11:115–29.

2. Wing L. Syndromes of autism and atypical development. In: Cohen DJ, Volkmar FR, eds. *Handbook of Autism and Pervasive Developmental Disorders*. 2nd edn. New York: Wiley, 1997:148–70.

3. Tantum D. The challenge of adolescents and adults with Asperger syndrome. *Child Adolesc Psychiatr Clin N Am* 2003;12:143–63.

4. Fombonne E. Epidemiological surveys of autism and other pervasive developmental disorders: an update. *J Autism Dev Disord* 2003;33: 365–82.

5. Howlin P. Outcome in high-functioning adults with autism with and without early language delays: implications for the differentiation between autism and Asperger syndrome. *J Autism Dev Disord* 2003;33:3–13.

6. Klin A, Volkmar FR. Asperger syndrome: diagnosis and external validity. *Child Adolesc Psychiatr Clin N Am* 2003;12:1–13.

7. Szatmari P, Bryson SE, Boyle MH et al. Predictors of outcome among high functioning children with autism and Asperger syndrome. *J Child Psychol Psychiatry* 2003;44:520–8.

8. Star E, Szatmari P, Bryson S, Zwaigenbaum L. Stability and change among high-functioning children with pervasive developmental disorders: A 2-year outcome study. *J Autism Dev Disord* 2003;33:15–22.

9. Tsatsanis KD. Outcome research in Asperger syndrome and autism. *Child Adolesc Psychiatr Clin N Am* 2003;12:47–63.

10. Ziatas K, Durkin K, Pratt C. Differences in assertive speech acts produced by children with autism, Asperger syndrome, specific language impairments, and normal developmental. *Dev Psychopathol* 2003;15:73–94.

11. Towbin KE. Strategies for pharmacological treatment of high functioning autism and Asperger syndrome. *Child Adolesc Psychiatr Clin N Am* 2003;12:23–45.

12. Emerich DM, Creaghead NA, Greather SM et al. The comprehension of humorous materials by adolescents with high-functioning autism and Asperger's syndrome. *J Autism Dev Disord* 2003;33:253–7.

13. Dahlgren S, Sandberg AD, Hjelmquist E. The non-specificity of theory of mind deficits: Evidence form children with communicative disabilities. *Eur J Cognitive Psychol* 2003;15:129–55.

14. Jansson-Verkasalo E, Ceponiene R, Kielinen M et al. Deficient auditory processing in children with Asperger syndrome, as indexed by event-related potentials. *Neurosci Lett* 2003;338:197–200.

15. Losh M, Capps L. Narrative ability in high-functioning children with autism or Asperger's syndrome. *J Autism Dev Disord* 2003;33:239–51.

16. Gardiner JM, Bowler DM, Grice SJ. Further evidence of preserved priming and impaired recall in adults with Asperger's syndrome. *J Autism Dev Disord* 2003;33:259–69.

17. Barton J. Disorders of face perception and recognition. *Neurol Clin* 2003;21:521–48.

18. Schultz RT, Gauthier I, Klin A et al. Abnormal ventral temporal cortical activity during face discrimination among individuals with autism and Asperger syndrome. *Arch Gen Psychiatry* 2000;57:331–40.

19. Hobson R, Ouston J, Lee A. What's in a face? The case of autism. *Br J Psychol* 1988;79:441–53.

20. Klin A, Jones W, Schultz R et al. Defining and quantifying the social phenotype in autism. *Am J Psychiatry* 2002;159:895–908.

21. Aldred S, Moore K, Fiztgerald M, Waring RH. Plasma amino acid levels in children with autism and their families. *J Autism Dev Disord* 2003;33:93–7.

22. Blacher J, Kraemer B, Schalow M. Asperger syndrome and high functioning autism: Research concerns and emerging foci. *Curr Opin Psychiatry* 2003;16:535–42.

23. Myles BS. Behavioral forms of stress management for individuals with Asperger syndrome. *Child Adolesc Psychiatr Clin N Am* 2003;12:123–41.

24. Safran SP, Safran JS, Ellis K. Intervention ABCs for children with Asperger syndrome. *Top Lang Disord* 2003;23:154–65.

25. Gerlai J, Gerlai R. Autism: a large unmet medical need and a complex research problem. *Physiol Behav* 2003;79:461–70.

26. Hollander E, Novotny S, Hanratty M et al. Oxytocin infusion reduces repetitive behaviors in adults with autistic and Asperger's disorders. *Neuropsychopharmacology* 2003;28:193–8.

Appendix – Generic and brand names of drugs

Generic names	US brand names	UK brand names
Drugs used in treatment		
Alprazolam	Xanax	Xanax
Bupropion	Wellbutrin	Zyban
	Zyban	
Buspirone	Buspar	Buspar
Chlordiazepoxide	Libritabs	Librium
	Librium	
	Mitran	
	Reposans	
Citalopram	Celexa	Cipramil
Clomipramine	Anafranil	Anafranil
Clonazepam	Klonopin	Rivotril
Dexamfetamine	Dexedrine	Dexedrine
	Dextrostat	
Diazepam	Valium	Diazemuls
		Diazepam Rectubes
		Stesolid
		Valclair
Fluoxetine	Prozac	Prozac
	Sarafem	
Fluvoxamine	Luvox	Faverin
Imipramine	–	Tofranil
Lorazepam	Ativan	Ativan
Mirtazapine	Remeron	Zspin
Nefazodone	Serzone	–
Oxytocin	Pitocin	Syntocinon
	Syntocinon	
Paroxetine	Paxil	Seroxat

Generic names	US brand names	UK brand names
Propranolol	Inderide	Inderal
		Syprol
Reboxetine	–	Edronax
Sertraline	Zoloft	Lustral
Venlafaxine	Effexor	Efexor

Drugs with potential for interactions

Procarbazine	Matulane	
Linezolid	Zyvox	Zyvox

Gaboxadol and pregabalin are in still in the development phase (page 49)

FAST FACTS

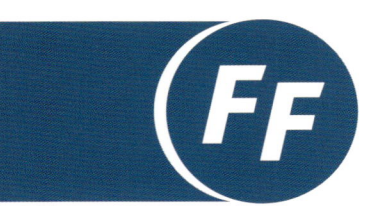

An outstandingly successful independent medical handbook series

Over one million copies sold

Written by world experts who are familiar with the latest and best research in their fields, these handbooks are:

- Concise and practical
- Right up-to-date
- Well structured for ease of reading and reference
- Copiously illustrated with useful photographs, diagrams and charts

Our aim for *Fast Facts* remains the same as ever: to be the world's most respected medical handbook series. As always, feedback on how to make individual titles even more useful is welcome (feedback@fastfactsbooks.com).

Some *Fast Facts* titles available

Acne
Allergic Rhinitis
Anxiety, Panic and Phobias
Asthma
Benign Gynecological Disease (second edition)
Benign Prostatic Hyperplasia (fourth edition)
Breast Cancer (second edition)
Brain Tumors
Chronic Obstructive Pulmonary Disease
Coeliac Disease
Colorectal Cancer
Contraception
Dementia
Depression
Diabetes Mellitus (second edition)
Diseases of the Testis
Disorders of the Hair and Scalp
Dyspepsia (second edition)
Eczema and Contact Dermatitis
Endometriosis (second edition)
Epilepsy (second edition)
Erectile Dysfunction (third edition)
Gynaecological Oncology
Headaches (second edition)
HIV in Obstetrics and Gynecology
Hyperlipidemia (second edition)
Hypertension (second edition)
Infant Nutrition
Inflammatory Bowel Disease
Irritable Bowel Syndrome (second edition)
Low Back Pain
Menopause
Minor Surgery
Multiple Sclerosis
Osteoporosis (third edition)
Prostate Cancer (fourth edition)
Prostate Specific Antigen (second edition)
Psoriasis
Respiratory Tract Infection (second edition)
Rheumatoid Arthritis
Sexually Transmitted Infections
Soft Tissue Rheumatology
Superficial Fungal Infections
Travel Medicine
Urinary Continence (second edition)
Urinary Stones

Forthcoming and recently published psychiatry titles

Fast Facts – Schizophrenia (second edition)
by Shôn W Lewis, Manchester, UK
and Robert Buchanan, Maryland, USA

Fast Facts – Anxiety, Panic and Phobias (second edition)
by Malcolm H Lader, London, UK and Thomas W Uhde, Detroit, USA

Fast Facts – Stress and Strain (second edition)
by James Campbell Quick, Texas, USA
and Cary L Cooper, Manchester, UK

Fast Facts – Specific Learning Difficulties
by Amanda Kirby, Cardiff, UK
and Bonnie J Kaplan, Calgary, Canada

Fast Facts – Parkinson's Disease
by Christopher G Clough, London, UK
Ray Chaudhuri, London, UK
and Kapil D Sethi, Georgia, USA

Fast Facts – Bipolar Disorder
by Guy Goodwin, Oxford, UK
and Gary Sachs, Boston, USA

Fast Facts – Sexual Dysfunction
by S Michael Plaut, Maryland, USA,
Alessandra Graziottin, Milan, Italy
and Jeremy PW Heaton, Ontario, Canada

Fast Facts – Depression (second edition)
By David S Baldwin, Southampton, UK
and Robert MA Hirschfeld, Texas, USA

Orders can be placed by telephone or via the website. For regional distributors or to order via the website, please visit www.fastfacts.com

For telephone orders, please call 01752 202301 (UK) or 1 800 538 1287 (North America, toll free)

For quotes for bulk orders (of 500 copies or more) please contact Sarah Redston at sarah@fastfacts.com

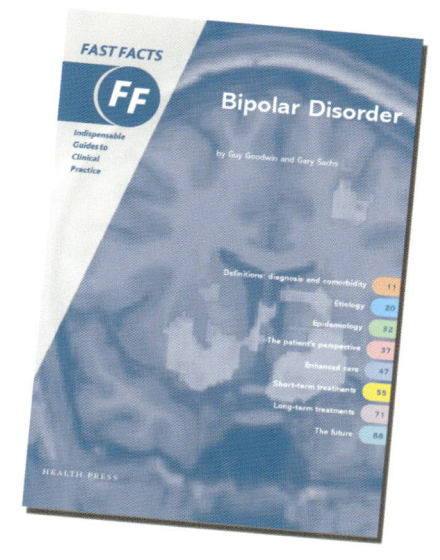

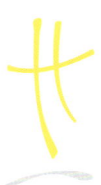

Health Press
medical publishing
at its best